THE ALL-RN
NURSING STAFF

THE ALL-RN
NURSING STAFF

Genrose J. Alfano, R.N., M.A., F.A.A.N.
Director, The Loeb Center for Nursing and Rehabilitation
Montefiore Hospital and Medical Center, Bronx, New York

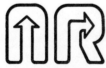

Nursing Resources
An information activity of Concept Development, Inc.
Wakefield, Massachusetts

Table of Contents

Contributing Authors

Genrose J. Alfano,
R.N., M.A., F.A.A.N.
Director
The Loeb Center for Nursing
and Rehabilitation
Montefiore Hospital and Medical
Center
Bronx, New York

Barbara J. Brown,
R.N., Ed.D., F.A.A.N.
Assistant Professor
Graduate Program in Nursing
Administration
Community Health Care Systems
School of Nursing
University of Washington
Seattle, Washington

Marguerite L. Burt,
R.N., B.S., M.P.H.
Chief, Nursing Service
Audie L. Murphy Memorial
Veterans' Hospital
San Antonio, Texas

Sylvia Carlson, R.N., M.S.
Associate Director
Nursing Education
Long Island Jewish-Hillside
Medical Center
New Hyde Park, New York

Luther Christman,
Ph.D., R.N.
Dean
College of Nursing and Allied
Health Sciences
Rush University
Chicago, Illinois

Alice L. Dahlen, R.N., M.S.N.

Director of Nursing Service
Meridian Park Hospital
Tualatin, Oregon

Barbara A. Donaho, M.A., R.N.

Corporate Director of Nursing
Sisters of Mercy Health Corporation
Farmington Hills, Michigan
(At the time this article was
written, author was Vice President
of Nursing, Abbott-Northwestern
Hospital Corporation, Minneapolis,
Minnesota)

Jean C. Forseth, R.N., B.S.

Medical Services Manager
Billings Deaconess Hospital
Billings, Montana

**Margaret L. McClure,
R.N., Ed.D., F.A.A.N.**
Executive Director of Nursing
Associate Administrator, University
Hospital
New York University Medical Center
New York, New York

Patricia W. Miller, R.N.

Administrator, Nursing
Eastern Maine Medical Center
Bangor, Maine

June Werner, R.N., M.S.N.

Chairman
Department of Nursing
Evanston Hospital Corporation
Evanston, Illinois

Preface

Those of us who are employed in hospital systems today are beset with pressures to reduce costs and simultaneously improve quality. Many cost-cutters argue that the objective is to reduce costs while maintaining the present system.

This argument is based on the fallacious assumption that the present system provides quality. That quality is lacking is evident from countless studies, from opinion polls of the public and of health care personnel, and from television and newspaper features, all of which have decried the depersonalization of care, the frequency of error, and the degree of staff incompetence.

These are some of the reasons that I believe make the use of ALL-RN nursing staff imperative. There are other reasons.

The use of assistive, adjunctive, nonprofessional personnel rather than RNs to carry out personal services, treatments, other procedures and overall supervision of daily patient care has resulted in fragmentation of care, duplication of effort, lack of accountability and more significantly, delayed recognition of changes in patient status.

I believe a team of persons functioning at different levels of competency in the same discipline ultimately reduces the level of performance to its lowest rather than its highest common denominator. We cannot afford to support such a team when a prepared competent nurse can perform the functions better, in less time, and usually *at less cost.*

The cost of delivering nursing service is directly related to the number of people who give the care, which in turn is directly related to the degree of competency and skill each possesses. Attempts by system managers and efficiency experts to reduce nursing care to a set of tasks, ranging from simple to complex, has only resulted in a more costly, less effective method of delivery.

Even though medical equipment, diagnostic procedures, and methods of treatment have become more costly and complex, personnel costs remain the highest cost factor in hospital budgets, and nursing services highest within that group. It becomes imperative then that we optimize the staff we have and the most effective way to do that is to ensure that we employ only well-prepared, good generalists, who are flexible and highly competent. This means professional nurses!

If there is an insufficient supply of professional nurses to staff hospitals today, it is only partially due to the reduced number of individuals graduating from educational programs. It is also due to the loss of so many prepared people to other occupational areas or to inactive status. But many of these people can be attracted back into the system when the level of quality improves the excitement and the reward that is so much a part of nursing, particularly in the care of the sick, return; in other words, when the practice of nursing is professional in its attitude and competence.

It is through the skills and acts of nursing (nurturing) that patients begin to regain strength and functional capacity. Professional nursing helps others to thrive and function using all their capacities, by supporting their life functions and by assisting them with acts they are unable to perform or have difficulty performing because of temporary or permanent incapacities. These acts may be integral to maintaining life, to enhancing life through alleviation of discomfort or expanding skills or capacities, or to healing or restoration of function. Nursing is based on sound and proven principles in the biophysical and social sciences. It draws on knowledge of growth and development, on concepts of maturation, and on an understanding of the interrelationship of living beings within the environment and society. *Nursing cannot be performed by persons who do not have this knowledge base.*

In July 1978, under the auspices of *Nursing Digest* (now *Nursing Dimensions*), a conference was held in Chicago to consider the concept of an ALL-RN staff for nursing care of hospitalized patients. The speakers chosen for that occasion were well recognized for their involvement with and support of this staffing concept.

For those of us who attended, it was a stimulating and exciting three days. In the following pages, we bring you some of the thoughts and ideas expressed at that meeting. It is particularly pertinent to study carefully the ALL-RN staff concept at this time, with the combined threat of reduced budgets and shortage of prepared nurses at the RN level.

We must no longer sacrifice patient care or the credibility of the importance of nursing in the recovery of the sick by allowing poorly prepared persons to deliver nursing care.

BIBLIOGRAPHY

Alfano, G. J. Healing or caretaking—Which will it be? *Nursing Clinics of North America,* 6:273-280, June 1971.

Hall, L.E. Nursing—what is it? *Canadian Nurse* 60(2): 150-154, 1964.

Henderson, V. *The Nature of Nursing.* New York: Macmillan, 1966.

The Advantages of the ALL-RN Nursing Staff

by Genrose Alfano

In order to fully appreciate the ramifcations of staffing mix or any staffing concerns related to an ALL-RN staff, we must consider the state of nursing today. We must decide what we want from nursing and a nursing service and what we think nursing must be. Over the thirty-five years of my career in nursing, we've moved toward a concept of nursing care that demands minimai knowledge, minimal skills, and minimal clinical competence. Juxtaposed with this view of nursing is the concept of professional nursing that demands rigorous clinical knowledge and assessment skills combined with decision-making ability. We have created a paradox in which *nursing care* requires minimal preparation and education but the *planning of nursing care* requires maximal preparation and education.

We have determined that professional responsibilities shall include patient advocacy, patient teaching, comfort, support and protection of patients, supervision of nursing care of patients, and collegial working relationships with other disciplines in the health-care system. Yet we remain uninvolved in the so-called mundane and simple tasks associated with the care of someone sick and someone dying, with the support of well-being and the prevention of illness. This we have decided to relegate or delegate to others. In fact, we do not even delegate any more, since delegation implies retention of some measure of responsibility. As things now stand even in the so-called new delivery system where we are attempting to regain our accountability through primary nursing systems, we still do not consider it necessary for a nurse to administer nursing care.

Perhaps I should clarify my notion of nursing care. Nursing care includes those measures that support comforting, that support health, growth, and welfare of individuals, that are most welcome in times of stress, in times of extreme discomfort, in times of extreme vulnerability. Such measures promote a renewal of self-worth. Performance of these measures demands skill and ability, not only in the technical components but also in the area of

1

interpersonal communication. Good nursing care is based on deliberate and supportive assistance, not the accidental, intuitive, well-meaning kind that on occasion can be almost as devastating as total absence of care.

DEFINING NURSING

Before discussing the advantages of an ALL-RN staff, we must review our definition of nursing. Presently, we seem better prepared to discuss what nursing is not. It is not medicine; we have duly advised the medical profession of that. It certainly is not physical therapy; we remain as far removed from the activities of the patients' daily lives as we possibly can. We rarely bathe them; we rarely move them from their beds; *and* we certainly do not feed them. Such a task can be performed by people who are less well-educated or well-prepared: occupational therapists teach patients how to eat; physical therapists teach patients how to retrain their muscles. We do not perform electrocardiograms; that duty belongs to an electrocardiographer. We have inhalation therapists who teach patients how to breathe and use various gases. Nursing is not bathing, feeding, and toileting. Neither is it taking temperatures, pulses, and respirations. That is data collection and nursing assesses data, it doesn't just collect it.

The picture I'm attempting to convey is that nurses have carefully identified all that they are not. There is very little left for them to be, except coordinators—and you've got to be careful about that because now there are unit managers.

We never delegated that duty to an aide or practical nurse: they were needed to give care. We had to do the "traffic managing." If that is the kind of nursing sevice we want, we don't need to discuss an ALL-RN staff. We do not need RNs at all. The only justification for preparing professional nurses is to improve the care of patients. We cannot continue to support nursing service systems in which ten people do what one well-prepared person could do in less time.

ADMINISTRATIVE ADVANTAGES OF AN ALL-RN STAFF

With an ALL-RN staff, less time and money are ultimately expended for training personnel on the job. Over the years, many nurses have suggested that most practical nurses are as good as, if not better than, RNs. The comparison is usually made between the practical nurse who has been with a particular unit for three to five years and a recently graduated, newly licensed RN who has just joined that unit. A new employee in a new situation, compared with an experienced employee working in the same setting over a long period of time, is bound to initially function less skillfully within that system.

If we only want staff members familiar with the rules and capable of functioning within a particular system as a result of their familiarity with that system, then we do not need an ALL-RN staff. We do not need professional nurses merely to carry out rules.

One can realize a cost savings by reducing the size of the staff. The best way to reduce staff is to employ more competent, adaptable people. Flexibility is really dependent upon knowledge, skill preparation, ability, and training. As Luther Christman has indicated, the more skilled the individual, the less "down time" and the less overall cost is incurred.

The administrative advantage of skilled personnel is that individuals who choose their profession are more likely to seek personal satisfaction through higher levels of career competence. Individuals who consider themselves "stuck with" their jobs are more likely to perform their functions at only the minimum level required. The more skilled the level of the group, the higher the level of quality. Group studies indicate that group performance will fall within its competency range, neither as good as the highest nor as bad as the lowest. Obviously, if you raise the lower level and increase the higher level, your median or quality performance increases.

From the standpoint of cost, LPNs generally command about three-fourths of the RN salary and the aides command two-thirds of the RN salary. Looking at these ratios and at the level of performance at which the RN is prepared, it is apparent that the RN is of greater value for the money expended.

We have developed a nursing system comprised of various fragmented tasks. Many of the individuals performing these tasks lack the necessary competencies for upgrading; others possess the skills but lack opportunities for growth. The question here is to what extent will administration provide opportunities for upgrading employees within its own setting? Certainly an end result would be a more satisfied employee group.

Another administrative advantage of an ALL-RN staff is the elimination of middle management. The less a system is fragmented, the less coordination is required. Some would suggest a reduction in top management as well, which certainly should give us pause. This view is consistent with nursing since we've maintained that if we really did a good job of nursing, we would work ourselves out of a job. Those of us in top levels of management might consider whether we want to do a good enough job to put ourselves out of a position. Perhaps at some point in time we will not have directors of nursing service, but clinical chiefs of nursing services who will offer their less-experienced colleagues the advice and wisdom of working with people rather than organizing timesheets and staffing patterns.

PATIENT ADVANTAGES OF AN ALL-RN STAFF

What are the advantages to the patient or the recipient of services of an ALL-RN staff? The increased capability of the RN to respond to the immediate concern of the patient is one principal advantage. At present, a patient concern that is not yet part of the treatment plan must be referred to the staff member in charge. That is called turnaround time or down-time. With an ALL-RN staff, the nurse can immediately respond to patient concerns. Consequently, the patient has the feeling that needs are being met in a timely manner, thereby reducing anxiety levels and promoting that much sought after "rest." Nurses who possess the clinical and scientific knowledge to understand what it is that they are observing can identify potential problems before they become critical or acute.

We have always maintained that a system in which the aides, LPNs, and other support staff reported to the RN was workable. One of my physician colleagues on the National Joint Practice Commission recently remarked that he thinks that it takes more skill to decide whether or not a problem exists than to find the solution to a problem. I'm not sure I agree with that statement, but I do believe that knowledge and skill are needed to identify a problem. Yet for years we have operated on the principle that our least prepared individuals collect the data upon which the most prepared make a judgment. No wonder the patients are so very anxious; they realize what is happening.

Recently a physician was notified in advance of an acute condition of a particular patient because the nurse who was working with the patient recognized that he was not his usual self. While vital signs varied only slightly, the total picture of that patient indicated from the nurse's assessment that he was beginning to get sick. Any of those individual symptoms collected and placed on a graph could have been ignored until the patient's condition reached an acute stage.

Educators emphasize the importance of patient education. Principles of learning suggest that individuals are more receptive to learning when they believe it to be something they wish to learn, when learning centers around their concerns and the goals of the learner. Learning is best reinforced when opportunities to apply new information exist in tandem with instruction. Following from these theories of learning, it is important that the nurse actually carry out all aspects of patient care so that teaching can occur while care is being given. This will avoid extended periods of time between patient care and the relevant patient education. Good nutrition can best be taught while feeding or assisting with meals. Then the patient is able to relate the rules of nutrition to the experience of eating a well-balanced meal. This is an immediate advantage to the patient.

Study of the behavioral sciences is firmly established in the nursing curricula, yet when nurses are placed in clinical situations they are not expected to draw upon this branch of knowledge; it is as though they were never exposed to the behavioral sciences. Some nurses complain about demanding patients. No one talks about a patient who feels deprived. The nurse who works directly with this patient has the opportunity to apply behavioral science principles. This allows the patient to understand her or his response to the environment without merely being told what to do and when to do it. Interestingly enough, if we help patients to examine their behavior, they will devise their own methods of coping that are more consistent with their own capabilities.

This approach also creates flexibility within the system. For many years, we have administered medicine in institutions without regard to the impact of the medication. Patients are released believing that TID medications must be taken at some magical daily interval, be it 9-1-5, 10-2-6, or 7-11-4. With an ALL-RN staff, there is no need for a medication nurse. We can begin to evaluate patient responses to medication. We can begin to help patients understand why medications are taken, when they should be taken, what responses to expect, and what modifications are possible. The more knowledgeable the care giver, the less restrained the patient.

Many patients are physically restrained because the care givers do not know how to cope with patient behavior. If we had knowledgeable people capable of coping with patient behavior and identifying patterns of behavior, we would be restraining less patients. We would not be tying elderly patients in bed at night for fear they would fall on the way to the bathroom. Observation of the time-period regularity of falls for such patients would almost certainly reveal a nightly pattern. With care givers on hand at the times indicated, there would be no need to restrain the patients.

We need to ask a major question. Why do our patients always need to go to the bathroom when we are not there? We should consider the advantages of an ALL-RN staff from that perspective. From an administrative standpoint, there would be fewer incident reports to sign. Administrative time would not be consumed solving problems that should not arise with a professional staff. Time could instead be devoted to long-range planning, research, and problem-solving in a more general vein with solution to such concerns as how we might eliminate restraints. Restraints are among the most inhumane aspects of the hospital environment.

IDENTIFYING THE RN DIFFERENCE

Lack of time is an assumed reality for most nurses. They will say they have no time to care for patients or to supervise aides and LPNs. Their time is devoted to collecting and disseminating bits of information. We assume that data are collected to formulate action. Actually, data are collected to be logged on the charts. Once data becomes entered on the charts, it is infrequent that care givers return to it for patient care. Without care givers in our systems who can act knowledgeably and deliberatively to intervene for and work with patients, who know that clinical entities suggest behaviors, or symptoms, who have the knowledge to work constructively with patients to regain their health, strength, and abilities, then we will not have the quality care we say we want. We will not have cost effective systems.

In addition, we will constantly be asked to cut down on our number of personnel. If we are unable to identify the RN contribution as distinct from that of the aide or the LPN, and if we continue to operate in a multi-level system, we will not utilize the full capabilities of the RN. My experience shows that multiple levels of personnel on a unit sharing goals and responsibilities result in division of tasks—this is my job and that is your job; people mark out their own territories. With only one level of personnel, there is no territorial demarcation.

The cost of hospitals is blamed to a large extent on medicine and nursing. Since nursing comprises the greatest number of personnel in nursing service, this is where cuts are expected. As long as we cannot demonstrate that the RN functions differently, we'll be asked to cut RN positions until we will end up with none, save an occasional supervisor. But we'll have an increase in on-the-job trainees which will set us back about forty years in nursing. After another ten years the system will discover that better preparation than on-the-job training is necessary so we'll send the trainees to school. Then we'll discover that they are too well educated to do nursing, and the cycle begins again.

The question is, can we stop it now? Do we believe that nursing is really important enough to require skill and preparation or do we believe as so many do, that is a manual, technical vocation; a series of isolated, independent tasks that can be taught on the job. There is no task that cannot be taught in about two weeks to one possessing some manual dexterity and a strong back. If that is what we believe nursing is, this conference is ludicrous. We don't need prepared people. I'm talking not about the registered nurse, but the individual prepared in professional nursing practice. That is supposedly what our Registered Nursing license ought to be. I might point out that having licensure for nursing in any state really doesn't matter. The level of entry for licensure is inconsequential as long as most of the nursing care is administered by unlicensed personnel.

Do we believe that nursing care is the most important discipline in the health-care system? If we believe that, we can then look at all these obstacles and work them out. We can be creative and innovative in helping people move laterally if they cannot administer professional nursing care and cannot be upgraded any other way. We can find ways of upgrading so that change does not mean an economic holocaust. We can return to nursing the status that it deserves as a professional discipline in the health-care system.

Audience: I must say as a nurse manager that I am quite concerned over recent inquiries as to whether the top administrator must be a nurse in nursing. I see myself as the chief clinician. I think I can still out-nurse most of my nurses, and basically I think that nursing managers must know what nursing is before we can expect our nursing professionals to carry on those things that you just defined.

Alfano: This is an issue that has arisen frequently. Many people believe that lay administrators are perfectly acceptable. If we want to go the route of clinical chief, I don't think we have a problem with whether or not a nurse is needed. If nursing believes, however, that its power is going to be in the area of administration, we had also better be prepared in administration if we're going to be nurse managers who have clinical competence plus administrative skills. Unfortunately too many nurses in the field of nurse management know little about administration. I'm not sure I knew much about administration when we started at Loeb. We must be better skilled in administration if we are going to justify the handling of large budgets and utilization of large numbers of personnel.

Audience: I am an assistant director of a hospital and director of nursing. My experience suggests that the changes need to start at the top. One of the things I've done is decentralize nursing as the first step toward a change to an ALL-RN staffing pattern. In place of supervisors, assistant directors of nursing, and so on around the shifts, each unit is headed by a nurse who is responsible for the clinical and administrative boundaries of the unit twenty-four hours a day, seven days a week. That doesn't mean, obviously, that the nurse is there at all times. The hours are flexible and there is no clocking; however, focusing responsibility and authority at the local unit level has been extremely effective. The staff nurses on the unit make patient-care decisions including overtime and numbers of nurses needed for given situations. We all know that nursing and patient needs change from week to week. I've found that the staff nurse's ability to assume more responsibility, which is the biggest issue, depends on the degree of authority, status, and importance given the nurse. There is much more money to position nurses at the local patient-care level where they are needed when some of these departments are decentralized. There are ways to preserve some of the important functions of central nursing through other structural mechanisms so that the baby isn't thrown out with the bath water, as it were.

Alfano: Decentralization is one choice, and thank you for pointing it out. It is interesting that when you expect people to live up to responsibility, they usually do it. Of course, the theory is that if you give people responsibility, you must allow them the authority to carry it out. I suspect that nursing administrators have moved to decentralization, especially as hospitals and institutions get larger and larger and the ability of the heads of departments to maintain meaningful contact with the ground level staff becomes more difficult.

Audience: I would like to comment on the statement that things must begin at the top. I'm a director of nursing and from what I've heard about primary care, I can't agree with that observation. Nursing management must support change, but it need not begin there. I think the most successful attempts have begun at the bottom and were supported at the top.

I'm looking at this in terms of primary nursing in my own facility. I am curious to know what strategies you use to trigger the thinking process and channel dissatisfaction toward implementing change through the nursing staff. The current desire for recognition among the staff nurses is an important trend for nursing management to note. I once believed that change could begin at the top, but I don't any more. Working together, supporting nursing as a whole, and recognizing the critical role of the staff nurse will promote more rapid and longer lasting change.

The other point I wanted to respond to is that of the nurse manager as an expert clinician. I don't believe that's realistic or practical. I also question the person who said that as a nurse manager she could run circles around her staff in providing care. At least that was my interpretation of what was said. I think my staff can run circles around me. I do believe, though, that as a nurse manager I am a professional person and have clinical expertise in evaluating and assessing what the staff is doing in terms of planning, identifying patient needs, and using solid nursing judgment. I can compete with my staff in nursing judgment and problem solving. In that respect I see a nursing manager as a clinician. At one time I skillfully started twelve to fifteen IVs each morning. I pity the patient who would be subject to my rusty technical skills now.

Alfano: Thank you. Certainly nursing is an applied science.

Audience: We get into fads administratively just as we get into fads educationally in almost every field. Direct and indirect care or the separation of applied skills from the judgmental process are totally artificial distinctions. As administrators, when we speak of centralization and decentralization, could we think in terms of the total system? At a medical center you are talking about the whole educational institution as well as a service to patients and acute-care center. There are, at the patient-care level, at the nursing-unit level, more legitimate authorities that must be dealt with, and nursing at the local level needs more than administrative support to effect change.

The whole process of effecting change involves unification of a department, different levels of authority to do different kinds of things. My practitioners with two years of clinical experience cannot compete with me for strategies to convince other disciplines, accountants, financiers, and the board of trustees about a whole new concept. I have an obligation to my staff; they should expect me to be at least five years ahead of them in the directions of professional nursing and patient care in the health-care system.

The practice of nursing, the technical skills are lost and can be regained but that isn't the whole story. It is integrating those skills and making instant decisions, while applying the skill simultaneously. We must consider the complexity of authority. We must avoid viewing the hierarchical structure as strictly negative and decentralization as the "in" thing, for we may end up being divided and conquered by the other sources of power that are more centralized and have a better means of intervention at the institutional level.

Audience: Given the different levels of RNs entering the field, how would you deal with those in an ALL-RN staff, assuming an inadequate supply of baccalaureate graduates and the necessity to utilize other levels?

Alfano: With our present licensure laws, you could probably use the nurses interchangeably. Registered nurses cannot be treated differently regardless of level of preparation. Presumably they are all prepared. They have all passed the same state boards and are licensed by their state to practice at a particular level of nursing.

From the standpoint of performance and drawing on my own personal experience, I have consistently found the baccalaureate nurse to be far and away the most professional person in terms of the performance of nursing care, given the opportunity to become familiar with the setting. The baccalaureate nurse is best able to integrate technical, clinical, behavioral, and physical activities; to view nursing as a process rather than a group of tasks to be completed within a specified period of time. I have found individuals from each of the other programs, the diploma program and the AD program, who have far surpassed their preparation and who became very good once they acquired the additional knowledge.

Nevertheless, all things being equal, certain knowledge must be gained formally as a foundation before people can really expand their thinking. We are constantly defending native intelligence, as opposed to formalized learning, when we should be developing native intelligence; developing it and formalizing it rather than defending it. We see a practical nurse that is very good and we defend practical nursing rather than imagining how good that practical nurse would be with more education and more skill. If we do develop criteria which differentiate competencies, we will no longer be able to use nurses with different educational preparation interchangeably. Some primary care centers are using the baccalaureate as the primary nurse and the AD as an associate. Registered nurses cannot be primary nurses until they have attained the baccalaureate degree. This is one method for working with different educational levels. In some places only the baccalaureate can assume the leadership role as a senior staff nurse; the AD does not assume that position without additional preparation.

We must attempt to change licensure laws. That will be a problem. Change does not occur without a certain amount of turmoil. We must consider which type of upheaval is of the shortest duration. If we continue with the present system, countless numbers of patients will suffer because we have failed to move to protect them by ensuring adequate care.

Audience: I would like to say something in defense of diploma nursing. I am a diploma nurse. I am going back to school to get my degree, but I find it unrewarding to some extent because they do not offer programs for us. I've been a nurse for approximately eleven years. I have grown in nursing. I believe in the current concepts of nursing, and I believe my knowledge has grown through independent learning. Colleges today are not geared to people such as myself. When I go back to school I would like to have my clinicals in an intensive care unit, coronary care unit, an intensive neonatal unit, because I have grown with nursing and I would like to learn the intensive part in more detail. To me probably the next four years will be a fantastic review which I do need and I'm sure we all need, but I still would like to learn more now rather than waiting until I have completed my four years for a masters.

Alfano: Yes, I think there is little doubt that whenever one changes from one system to another, people get caught in the middle. The diploma nurses have certainly gotten caught in the middle of a system in which the baccalaureate programs have decided not to grant credit for what has happened to the diploma nurse and have merely presented that person with another general program. There is a program in New York State called the Regent's External Degree. Those of you who believe you have the knowledge comparable to any baccalaureate graduate today, even though you did not graduate from a baccalaureate program, are welcome to take these exams. If you pass, you will be conferred a degree by a very reputable university. You will have a baccalaureate that is worth a baccalaureate. If you are already licensed in your state, you don't have to worry about licensure.

One of the obstacles in nursing that has prevented us from moving forward is that each of us has areas which we feel we must defend. Many people in this room, including myself, are diploma graduates. I think that I did get a trial-by-fire type of education. I also didn't learn an awful lot, and a lot of what I learned, I learned by happenstance, not deliberately.

We don't need to defend the past anymore. What we must do is examine what we have, why it isn't working the way it ought to, and how we can make things better.

I don't think it matters whether we are nurse managers or clinical chiefs, if in the process of running a nursing service we facilitate better patient care and better quality care. I don't think it matters whether we decentralize or centralize, if our system works so that patients receive better care and nursing care is at the level and quality that we want it to be. We must set aside our own personal hurts and traumas and look at the problem rather than try to explain why it exists.

I agree that nursing, if it's going to change, must have support, must have wisdom. The nature of the system does not matter; what matters is whether the system promotes good patient care. To do this we need formally prepared, knowledgeable, committed, professional people who are taking care of others where they are most vulnerable, most at risk, most in need of help in preserving their sense of themselves and their dignity. If we have that will we have made a large stride forward in nursing care.

Experiences of Setting Up an ALL-RN Staff

by Barbara J. Brown

In September of 1973, Family Hospital, Milwaukee, Wisconsin, was a less than ordinary community hospital facility comprised of 220 acute-care and 174 extended-care beds. How do you attract, recruit, and retain staff at all for a private community hospital in a city that has over 500 staff RN vacancies between 24 major hospitals? These were highly competitive hospitals; medical center, teaching center hospitals. How do you even get nurses, much less dream of or think of an ALL-RN staff? How do you innovate nursing in order to excite nurses so much that they want to come into this nonprofessional setting? These were some of the questions that I had to ask myself with administration at the hospital to decide what we were going to do and how we were going to do it.

At the time, the nursing staff included 62 permanent full-time and part-time RNs, 120 NAs, and 35 LPNs. There were clear violations of safe nursing-care standards, including the delegation of RN functions to LPNs. Many of the staff had been hired with no commitment to work evenings, nights, or weekends. Temporary agency nurses were employed to work regularly and in such key positions as night supervision.

How could nurses with different educational preparations possibly be attracted to that environment? I wondered how I could even stay there when I learned what nursing practice was.

How do you go about organizing a nursing service for nursing care with an ALL-RN staff? What can you do to change it? To change direction, nurses had to be accountable, twenty-four hours a day, seven days a week and there had to be some major recruitment goals. It was easy to establish them, but to attain them was a different thing. The specifics of the recruitment program are available in the *American Journal of Nursing*[1]. Attracting nurses may be possible in any setting; however, the setting must be attractive to retain them,

13

and this required changes in nursing practice.

INITIATING CHANGE

The first step toward change is goal setting. We began by asking ourselves what we believed in about this hospital, its mission in the community, and what role would be played by nursing. Our conclusions prompted our renaming the hospital to Family Hospital in the spring of 1974. To translate the statement of family-centered care into reality, change had to occur at every level, including the board of trustees, the medical staff, and the nursing staff.

How is nursing and the total patient-care system organized to accomplish this? It begins with recognition of patient and family needs that must be defined. Family is defined as any significant person the patient deems appropriate, not necessarily related by blood or marriage. The system had to be sensitive to involving significant others. They could then participate with the patient in determining the health-care needs. The patient and family's right to control their own lives and participate in decisionmaking to the greatest degree possible was an accepted premise. Patient and families were considered members of the health team. We had a responsibility to assist them with support at home, and encourage them to participate wherever possible in their own care. Nursing and other patient care services are responsible for the assessment, planning of care, teaching, coordinating and evaluating in collaboration with physicians toward discharge planning. The physician focuses on diagnosis and treatment.

Having defined the family-centered care model as direction for change, nursing's mission became clear. If we believed in family-centered care for our patient population, only the RN in the nursing care system could provide it. The RN had to be the care giver. The reason our hospital exists and any hospital exists is for nursing care. If a physician did not need nursing care for his patients, twenty-four hours a day, seven days a week, would that patient be admitted to our hospitals and to our extended-care facilities? The patient would not. He would be treated through ambulatory care.

PROFESSIONAL NURSING DOCUMENTATION

The environment for professional practice of nursing is organized through creation of a system that clearly mandates the role of the RN. Patient and client needs are identified using a formalized documentation system. This requires that the RN and no other person, implement the nursing process. The RN is responsible for documenting the nursing history, the patient-care plan, daily activity and clinical data specific to the patient, and patient progress notes from the nursing perspective.

Nurses and physicians document progress notes sequentially in the same chart form in order to communicate both nursing and medical observations pertinent to the patient's change in condition or progress. When the RNs realized their professional responsibility for recording nursing process on the patient's chart, they decided that additional LPNs should not be hired. That decision, while a long time in the back of my mind, came not from me but from the staff nurses themselves, who said, "We'll last, just get us more RNs; we're not going to run scared about shortages; we're going to get through."

NURSE INTERNSHIP PROGRAM

More RNs meant hiring new graduates. What do we do about all these new practitioners entering practice? These nurses, prepared in associate degree, diploma, and baccalaureate programs are being expected to do something in a care system that they can't do. Learning by fire usually leads to the "burned out" nurse syndrome. Regardless of the educational background, every nurse has a right to expect a transition into practice. Nursing services have systems of care expecting twenty-four hour accountability, seven days a week, with a nursing knowledge base enabling implementation of the family-center care model. New graduates need a transitional program. A three-month internship program was developed with night and evening experience included in the curriculum. Operating room experience was included as a means of learning aseptic technique. It was offered as an elective experience first and every new graduate opted to take it. The nurse epidemiology studies indicated that the aseptic control levels of nursing practice in Ob-Gyn, postsurgical, medical were enhanced considerably. The gaps between service and education were bridged and a patient-care value system was created. Obviously, nurses giving patient care attracted nurses.

The new graduates were protected from nights and evenings until they developed sufficient clinical decision-making experience to assume knowledgeable, competent, twenty-four hour accountability. Courses on history-taking and physical diagnosis were taught so that the nursing staff could assume responsibility for the total assessment of patient needs in a partnership relationship with medicine.

JOINT CHARTING

Problem-oriented charting was taught to the nurses. A trial unit was established to demonstrate succinct, precise progress note recording, and to integrate the nurse and physician progress note recording. When the JCAH cited the new documentation system on the trial unit as an improvement, the medical records committee, the medical executive committee, and the medical staff accepted nurse/physician progress note recording.

The role of the registered professional nurses evolved in an exciting way. If one promotes an ALL-RN staff, does it mean you're really going to promote an environment for professional practice? Are you going to have a practice model that will allow nurses to reach and stretch every bit of what professionalism is all about?

What about the role of the nurse practitioner?

NURSE PRACTITIONER ROLE

There are distinct differences between medical care and nursing care. An example of this distinction occurred in the treatment of sexual assault victims in a way that was sensitive, caring, and comprehensive.

In the initial development of the study, the district attorney was asked, "Why can't a nurse be primary care giver—the full implementation of the RN—in assessing wellness data and collecting evidence?" Is it necessarily a medical function to collect specimens? Is it necessarily doing a wellness assessment of a patient who usually doesn't even have a need for medical intervention but needs sensitive crisis intervention, preferably by someone who is of the same sex? There is nothing more demeaning to a rape victim, after being assaulted by a male, than to be set up in stirrups while waiting for the male gynecologist to arrive. This situation is handled with a great deal of sensitivity by many fine physicians but the nurse could play a critical role in giving care to the patient.

Two years after the start of the Sexual Assault Treatment Center (SATC), the police department and the district attorney asked for a trial period using the nurse practitioner to collect the evidence. Cost was the major reason. The police had to wait an hour while the MD was responding to the call to evaluate the victim. This was taking too much down-time for the police. If the nurse could take care of the victim, time would be reduced. Today physicians are called in for patients who are under thirteen years of age or where there is a need for medical intervention. The nurse practitioner role came into its own in this acute-care setting on the gynecological unit. Nurses need professional role implementation in an ALL-RN setting.

PROFESSIONAL ACCOUNTABILITY

A formal hierarchical, traditional, supervisory structure was changed to one of unit participatory management where every staff nurse participates in budget definition, number of patient-care hours needed, the patient classification need indexes, and determination of unit goals. The decentralized management system took four years to develop the staff nurses to the point where they could be sensitive to patient quality care needs and the indices they needed to manage those needs. They even volunteered off a unit because "their census was down and they were overstaffed" based on their criterion for patient-care need indices, for patient-care hours, and their budgetary goals for the unit.

They were professionally accountable, not only for the twenty-four hour care for their patients but for the organization and its cost effectiveness. The management process and development of the staff nurse clinical decision-making skills were key change factors. Having a peer review system that rewards nurses for excellence in practice rather than for hierarchical movement in an organization is essential to professional growth. Those nurses who are fully accountable for patient case loads should be eligible for the highest level competency. Therefore, a combination of accountability for twenty-four hour management, planning, giving of care, patient case load, and the clinical knowledge base leads to a professional decentralized peer review system. This is the environment that needs to be created to organize and foster an ALL-RN staff for professional nursing practice.

REFERENCES

1. Brown, J. How to succeed in recruiting. *American Journal of Nursing,* 1976, 76 (4),604.

Accountability with an ALL-RN Nursing Staff

by Luther Christman

Concern has been voiced for humanitarian treatment of persons who are being displaced in the change to an ALL-RN staff. This is easily accomplished, given that the positions have existed for many years, but the turnover is enormously high. There is no long-term commitment to nursing for many of the personnel in such positions. Turnover varies with the state of the economy: when it's brisk outside, no one wants the jobs; when it's poor outside, they'll take them. Nationwide data support these trends.

Regarding the issue of cost effectiveness, the studies that Richard Jelinek and I conducted at a major university, which were later replicated at Rush, showed that aides are the most expensive worker in the nursing department, particularly when one measures cost per unit of care rather than remuneration per hour. In our study at two different hospitals, aides average 25 percent unoccupied time in the course of the day because they are not self-directed. Nurses average 8 percent unoccupied time which is much less than the unoccupied time for women workers generally, who average about 15 percent unoccupied time. In addition to that, we found that aides spend 25 percent of their day receiving information, under supervision, or instruction by a nurse. Most investigators before us labeled that as occupied time. We took the position that it was unoccupied time. Without the aides, the time would not be spent. We then looked at the effect of this expenditure of nursing time. If the aides were spending 25 percent of their time receiving instruction, nurses had to be spending 25 percent of their time in instructing. Taking the two 25 percent periods of unoccupied time in aides implies that it takes two aides to do one full-time job in the course of the day. This is much more expensive than employing a nurse with a master's degree.

Considering that nurses spend 25 percent of their time instructing, it takes five nurses to do the work of four with aides present. These data do not even touch upon the high cost of aide training at full salary with costly instructors and enormously high turnover. Turnover kills any budget. That is just a

19

beginning; I will only mention the data that Georgopoulos and I accumulated, suggesting that it would be cheaper to staff a hospital with every nurse having master's degree than any other staffing.

You may wish to examine a simulation that Richard Jelinek and I did in the mid-'60's. Looking at nursing activities, we had previously found that 75 percent of the time of each nurse in the population studied was spent in nonclinical activities during the course of a day. We projected these figures in the simulation to the 7600 hospitals then in existence in the United States. We found that if nurses restricted themselves to clinical activities—just patient care in the primary nursing mode—we would have had enough nurses (given perfect distribution) to fully staff every hospital in the United States with an ALL-RN staff. These findings died in the hands of most nurse directors and hospital administrators. The research was published in an article but received very little response. There were nationwide indications of growing interest in an ALL-RN staff and these findings were included in a popularized article in *Saturday Review of Literature.* For those who want to know more specifically about the move at Rush from a staff of 1200 people of which only 25 percent were RNs to what we have today, the data are reported in an article in *Nursing Digest.*

Continuity of care has long been a major theme in the nursing literature. Continuity of care, however, demands responsible behavior that is highly visible and constantly present. Thus, it has as a basic requisite a built-in pattern of accountability. Gaber and Franklin[1] state that accountability exists whenever there is delegation of authority or responsibility. As used, accountability refers to the extent to which an entity, person, group, or organization is liable and responsible for its performance. While accountability and responsibility are synonymous, Greenfield notes that responsibility preceeds accountability[2].

The normative structure of nursing departments provides a means of determining the level of accountability each is striving to attain. Too often the manner in which care is given and the staffing pattern mix are structural impediments to accountable behavior. Professional and ethical commitments to responsible clinical practice are greatly curtailed if team or functional nursing is the chief organizational device for the management of patient care.

The social structure components of the organization along with the knowledge systems of the participants in the organization are the most significant indicators of the behavior of all persons in the organization. For too long attention has focused on personality characteristics. Those who managed departments of nursing were preoccupied with human relations training. They attributed communication breaks to the idosyncratic behavior of individuals and explained failures in the nursing care system in terms of personality shortcomings. Such orientations to management are subtly seductive and easy to embrace because they establish a form of blame avoidance and facilitate the use of scapegoating to excuse managerial failures.

Contrast this approach to the utilization of primary nursing as the organizing motif for nursing care. Theoretically, the structure is organized so that the concept of perfect accountability dominates all the organizational arrangements. This concept is equally applicable to all levels of the organization from the staff nurse to the chief nursing executive, although it is highlighted by the nurse/patient alignment. When this alliance is in its best form, every error of commission and omission in nursing can be traced unerringly to each respective nurse. But the other side of the coin is equally revealing—so can every effective intervention that facilitates the recovery of the patient. Thus, the general competence of each nurse can be assessed and progress toward increased competence can be noted more easily.

The type and amount of knowledge between an ALL-RN staff and mixed classes of nursing personnel are readily contrasted. It is easy to build accountability in the former and awkward, if not impossible, to build it in the latter. Standards of care are a one-to-one correlative of the mix of staff. In one, the full professional role can be utilized to achieve desired standards, but the other must depend on task specialization with all its accompanying intraorganizational strain to achieve acceptable standards. Even under the best of conditions, this must result in less than professional care because that level must be empirically consistent with the amount of training possessed by the persons administering direct patient care. Thus, the higher the ratio of registered nurses to others on the staff, the greater the probability of approaching a professionally desirable level of performance.

EXPLORING DIFFERENCES IN LEVELS OF ACCOUNTABILITY

Some contrasting concepts may explain differences in the levels of accountability. The first is diffuse responsibilities versus specific responsibilities. In team nursing, it is almost impossible to pinpoint responsibility. Patients are more likely to be cared for by routine procedures, policies, and rules than by the canons of science. Nurses seem to be present to make the organization look good instead of aiding patients. Under primary nursing, patients are managed through assessment, monitoring, and advocacy. In addition, a necessary prerequisite for the growth of ethical considerations of care is a design of care that emphasizes accountability.

The second set of contrasting concepts are complete responsibility versus particularized responsibility. Complete responsibility means that the authority and accountability are decentralized down to each individual nurse for the set of patients that are specifically allocated to his or her care. In particularized responsibility, each person is allocated a set of tasks that usually are rotated daily among members of the staff. This form of task specialization has been used as an avoidance mechanism to escape individual accountability and to spread the responsibility across a large number where it becomes almost impossible to monitor. It is self-evident that responsibility can be precisely allocated if all the staff nurses are registered nurses.

The third concept is continuous versus discontinuous patient assignment. If a nurse is assigned to the same patients during their hospitalization and is accountable for the quality of their nursing outcomes, a different order of behavior is expressed than in situations in which tasks and patients are rotated daily. The quality of performance of each nurse can be more variable and unnoted when there are discontinuous relationships with patients.

The fourth concept is a contrasting of relationships with physicians. These can either be professional-colleague or physician-dictate in their texture. In primary nursing, the same nurse and the same physician are collaborating daily for the welfare of their patients. It is out of this endeavor over many patients that collegial relationships evolve. In a mixed nursing staff where team nursing predominates, physician-dictate behavior is more evident. When physicians are uncertain both as to whom is caring for their patients and the qualifications of the nursing-care providers, they then are more prone to use their authority to write orders as the chief means of communicating with the nursing staff. Thus, social and professional distance occurs with all its accompanying emotional overtones. Patients, physicians, and nurses are all dissatisfied. Legal compliance is more evident than professional zeal and excitement.

The fifth concept is individual legal vulnerability as opposed to organization vulnerability. In a staff composed only of registered nurses, it is possible to stimulate the growth of individual commitment to ethical and legal concerns. Nurses cannot experience this growing edge unless they have a consistent and primary relationship with patients. When team nursing is utilized, the tendency towards sterile legalism is greatly increased, instead of monitoring care to ensure that no ethical or legal breaks happen to patients.

Lest it be assumed that the burden of proof is on the staff nurse, we should examine the accountability of top and middle managers. The chief nurse executive is responsible for ensuring that nursing activity includes only that which can be defined as clinical. Nonclinical activities detract time and interest from the clinical enterprise and should be the responsibility of other departments embraced by the patient support services. Directors of nursing must be certain that this proper allocation of work takes place. In addition, the establishing of centers of care, quality assessment and control, a salary reward system acting as an economic incentive to stimulate the development of clinical competence, adequate budgets, and the creation of an organizational climate serving as a growth media for broadening and amplifying the expressive and instrumental roles of nurses, are responsibilities that cannot be avoided.

As a capstone to all these organizational variables, it will be necessary for nurses to begin to function under a form of self-government similar to that used by university faculty and attending physician staffs to bring responsibility and accountability to sophisticated levels. When nurses participate in peer review, in limiting practical privileges, in monitoring practice, enforcing standards of nursing care, and similar activities, then and only then will they be fully accountable and fully professional. Since professional status is tied to the quantity and quality of these forms of activities, it appears that staffs composed only of registered nurses can achieve the level of accomplishment needed to manage full or perfect accountability.

REFERENCES

1. Christman, L. and Jelinek, R. Old patterns waste half the nursing hours. *Modern Hospitals* 108(1):78-86, 1967. See also Christman, L. Role of nursing in organizational effectiveness. *Hospital Administration* 13(3):40, 1968.
2. Christman, L. Would a stewardess help? *Saturday Review,* Feb. 4, 1967, 65-67.

Established Role Definitions for Nurses and Support Personnel

by Barbara Donaho

Whether viewed as an obstacle or a challenge, established role definitions for nurses and support personnel exist in most hospital organizations. These definitions, regardless of their relation to actual practice, affect the viability of a change to an ALL-RN staff. The issue of a rigidly defined job description must be dealt with in the context of change. Beyond that, one must look to strategies for implementing change.

I am presently in the process of merging three very individual hospitals into one consolidated corporation. This merger began in 1970; when I came to the setting in 1975, there had never been a meeting of any of the nursing staffs or leadership of these three facilities. While they were all part of a corporate structure, there was no exchange among them regarding such matters as philosophy of care. In fact, they operated in competition to one another with different organizational philosophies and job functions. I was recruited to create a corporate department of nursing in that organization. During my first year, the decision was made to consolidate the buildings onto one campus. Clearly the day was coming when three different operations and sets of performance expectations could no longer exist.

We managed to develop a statement of our philosophy that met the approval of all three departments. Within that framework we defined an organizational structure that would lead to a corporate department. Since September of 1975, I have grappled with many of the concepts and strategies of change and with change as a process. As we focus on change as a process, we must recognize it as a stranger to our environment; as something we have not previously experienced.

THE PROCESS OF CHANGE

Some of the issues surrounding change can be identified through the experience of others, yet it is comforting to know that the process of change has

25

been the subject of numerous studies. We need not rely solely on gut feelings.

Arnold J. Toynbee, author of *Change of Habit and the Challenge of Our Times,* is one such authority. There is much in his book that is appropriate to nursing because we as a profession are very much tied to tradition. Toynbee states at the outset that most people are not moved to peer any further into the future than is required for present practical purposes when life seems satisfactory and secure. We live day by day. We become acutely concerned with the future beyond the horizon of the present only when the times are out of joint and the prospect of the future looks menacing to us.

In nursing, the future is rather frightening, given the pressures on the health care industry. In my particular setting, the HSAs are well under way and very effective. The Metropolitan Health Board in conjunction with the Citizens' League recently decided to close 3000-4000 hospital beds within the next three years and they have identified some of the hospitals that they think should be closed. Translate this occurrence to your own setting and imagine the response from the community and professionals.

Toynbee goes on to say that in the arena of human affairs, experience enables us merely to guess. We are dealing with human beings, which inhibits our ability to plan for and control the process of change. We can use history, we can use the knowledge we possess about individuals and human nature, but sometimes we forget that humans do have the option of choosing. Those of us committed to a choice of primary nursing with an ALL-RN staff must ensure that our staffs are informed of their rights and the choices available to them. If they are not part of that initial decision making and if they do not support it, they will find ways to impede the direction that we deem appropriate for them. If we begin to explore options with our staffs and listen to them, we may uncover some options that were previously overlooked. We as nurse leaders do not have all of the answers, and I do not think we should.

STABLE INGREDIENTS IN HUMAN NATURE

Returning to Toynbee for another reference, he has identified four stable ingredients in human nature which are relevant to nursing. For the focus of this discussion, I will cite three of Toynbee's ingredients and substitute my own for the fourth.

The first ingredient is consciousness, both of self and of the universe outside of oneself. One of our greatest challenges is to increase the level of consciousness or awareness of nurses toward their environment and its effect upon them. I have found the staff in all three divisions of my present setting to be unaware of societal changes or governmental pressures, whether national or local, until they hit the front page of the newspaper. We have a responsibility to educate or to broaden the awareness of our staffs, for their increased consciousness can only positively affect the nursing profession.

The second ingredient is the will to choose, which derives from our consciousness revealing the possibility of choice. If the professionals are educated and conscious, they do have some choices. We cannot forget that some may choose to have no part of change. But for as many people as we lose, we may retain like numbers who have almost reached the point at which they don't see nursing as a profession. They may remain in the system if we can get to them. When we begin to raise their level of consciousness, they will realize that they are professionals and do not only have the right but the responsibility to make some choices.

The third ingredient that Toynbee identifies is human recognition of the distinction between good and evil. It has often been said that when we expect the best of our staffs, they will perform with flying colors. Unfortunately, we in nursing tend to subscribe wholeheartedly to a certain modality; we define one modality as good and another bad. We label our staffs good or bad depending on their adherence to a given modality. If we can begin to recognize differences of opinion and discuss issues without personal attack or labeling, we will move toward change through the involvement of the staff.

Toynbee, as I indicated, identifies one other ingredient, but I have substituted an ingredient of my own, that of curiosity, which I feel is more pertinent to our discussion. Curiosity is essential in realizing the range of available options and in stimulating creativity. It can lead the staff to investigate and explore their options. If we convince our staffs that we are interested in what they think and if we empathize with their points of view rather than condemn them, they will indeed emerge in creative force. When we establish an advisory committee and purposely plan not to heed its advice, our action becomes window-dressing and the staff is quick to recognize it as such. When we can give the members of our staffs the option of learning from their own mistakes in an environment that accommodates the making of some mistakes, they will continually try and will progress. If we condemn and desert them, they will make no effort to broaden the bases of their experience.

One of the major changes in the health-care system that has a great impact on nursing is the voice of the consumer. If we believe that patient needs should be identified by patients and that we should be responding to them, we must recognize consumer input and assume the role of advocate for the consumer. Recently the clinical director of nursing responsible for obstetrics and gynecology met with a couple interested in making arrangements for a delivery utilizing our birthing room facilities. By previous history this was the woman's fourth pregnancy; her previous pregnancies were terminated with C-sections. The couple wanted to handle the entire birthing process on their own; neither wanted the pregnancy to end as the others had. They met with our staff to formulate and write a contract for care. This contract for care was not the first one written so that in itself posed no problem to the staff. The woman advised the staff that she wanted no nurse present during delivery; she only wanted the staff available as a back-up. She and her husband would deliver the baby entirely on their own. The staff recognized the couple's rights as consumers but were very concerned with their responsibility as nurses and decided that what the couple wanted and the care they felt should be provided had to be negotiated. We in nursing tend to think of negotiation as a labor-union tactic having no place in the matters of nurses or patients. This is naive and can on occasion be foolhardy.

The staff advised the couple that they could not accept their conditions for delivery under the circumstances and suggested that they review the matter together—the risks, the pros and cons, what the couple wished to gain from this experience. Together they arrived at a solution agreeable to both sides. By talking, negotiating, and reaching accord whether between consumer and staff or staff and staff, we can begin to respond to the consumer, we can respond to our own sets of expectations.

Citizen groups are moving toward more collective action. Community groups are questioning the heights of buildings, provisions for emergency room services, the nature of ambulatory care, and the degree of support which can be expected from the hospital as the health-care provider for the community. Governmental regulations are a major factor in their control and input. A new, more frequently heard external source is the legal voice or court decision. I think we will be faced with increasingly more clearly defined accountabilities through the courts. Whether we will be moving with it, ahead of it, or behind it depends on how we define our own role within nursing. We can all give due recognition to technology, what that is doing for us and how it is forcing change, how it forces us to even modify the process from time to time as we are trying to keep up with it. The changes in life are the essence of life. But they can be anxiety producing and for that reason we must consider our response to change.

HUMAN RESPONSES TO CHANGE

Incumbent with change is risk which often becomes an obstacle to action because people fear failure—the plan may not work, we may not be able to do what we want. This can have long-range impact on people. They may be unwilling to try again unless different support systems are introduced. Our ability to act is influenced by whether we allow mistakes to be equated with failure or with learning.

The change process itself will be costly. It is foolhardy to fail to identify and plan for costs in advance or to fail to build evaluation of the process into the strategy for implementing change. We must also recognize the challenge of dealing with physical and mental strain during the process of change, particularly on the leadership. Head nurses, clinicians, or supervisors may be challenged or bucked, may be verbally or nonverbally abused because of changes. There must be reinforcement for the validity of the direction taken, otherwise many will despair and want to back off.

The last risk that I wish to mention is union resistance to change. The issue of job security will surely be raised by the unions and we must be in a position to validate the benefits of change. We must look closely at our job descriptions. These affect not only nursing but every department that intersects nursing. You cannot easily change details of job descriptions whether concerning accountabilities or functional points of the nursing process that do not affect other services. If the rationale for change isn't understood or accepted, if there is a threat to territorial prerogative, you have come full circle to the issue of altering staff behavior in actual terms rather than just on paper. If barriers are too great or if the abuse from other departments is too great, the staff will say, "well, it's only a job description," and change is halted.

First and foremost we must begin to develop strategies to change behavior, to advance the staff from a task to a process orientation. We might be advised to think in terms of the obstacles to using the nursing process because that is what our job description should be based on.

REFERENCE

1. Brown, J. How to succeed in recruiting. *American Journal of Nursing*, 1976, 76 (4), 604..

Reports of the Work Groups Identifying Obstacles of the ALL-RN Nursing Staff

by Genrose Alfano, Marguerite Burt, Luther Christman, Barbara Brown, June Werner, Margaret McClure, Barbara Donaho, and Sylvia Carlson

Burt: With such a provocative and stimulating group, I didn't have to work hard at all—for which I'm most grateful. Our group chose the following obstacles, which I list not in any order of priority.

(1) Inadequate recruitment of RNs to staff health care facilities.

(2) Stability and tenure of aides and LPNs resulting in low turnover within these groups.

(3) Power of organized labor within both the nonprofessional groups and in many of the professional nurse groups.

(4) Lack of true professionalism in many areas of nursing.

(5) Resistance to change by administrators, particularly in phasing out the nursing assistant and LPN positions.

(6) Resistance to change by the medical staff, some of whom view the expanded role of nursing as a threat.

One member of the group shared the experience of the doctor whom, during a coffee break with the administrator, says, "Oh, you know those nurses." While they're encouraging our efforts to be professional—a true member and colleague—many are also undermining us when our backs are turned.

(7) Inadequate promotion for the nurse as a direct provider of care, particularly when we talk about the cost of the RN.

(8) Inadequate definitions of the nursing function. As mentioned yesterday, we often speak of what nursing isn't instead of what nursing is.

(9) Political clout of the nonprofessional. Similarly, discrepancy in funding of LPN schools versus professional schools of nursing.

(10) Nurses' own attitudes toward the role of the RN and commitment to total patient care. Some nurses would prefer that others assume certain patient-care responsibilities rather than nursing assuming responsibility for total patient care.

(11) Inadequate or nonexistent support services. This obstacle was repeat-

edly mentioned. Even with support services, nursing seems to pick up the slack in their absence. As we talked about this, one member of our group remarked that she would be satisfied just to eliminate passing the dietary trays. As we explored further, we concluded that really we aren't talking about just passing the trays. We are talking about setting up the trays, putting food on the trays, and so on. Lack of support services must be addressed when we talk about the cost of professional nursing.

(12) Third party reimbursement. We thought this will continue to be an obstacle to many of us until a definitive statement is made on, for instance, the patient's bill which specifies nursing costs.

(13) Lack of valid nursing standards.

(14) Questionable validity of our tools for measuring quality of care.

(15) Place of nursing in the organizational hierarchy. In short, the power structure.

(16) Shortage of qualified faculty and nursing administrators. We were fortunate to have one group member with a background in nursing service and in education, who shared her experiences in nursing education. We need a cross-section of people like her who can articulate our goals. We need qualified faculty who can practice nursing and nurse administrators who can facilitate that practice. In a similar vein, lack of collaboration on the preparation of the nurse between faculty and administrators is another obstacle in educating our nurses. This is a long-standing complaint heard everywhere we go.

(17) Political naivete. We lack knowledge of obtaining and using power.

(18) Ill-conceived design of our facilities. We brainstormed about architectural designs and admonished ourselves to become involved in the areas where nursing will be practiced.

(19) Lack of tangible rewards for good clinical performance. In this context, the Peter Principle was noted.

(20) Involving the physician in planning of medical care. This obstacle was discussed at some length.

(21) Lack of coordination of non-nursing activities falling within the realm of nursing.

(22) Our unwillingness to accept failure.

(23) Lack of creativity at times within nursing itself. We saw this as an obstacle that we would like to have challenged.

Alfano: Thank you for that list of obstacles. There are days when you wonder if you really can succeed at all!

In all probability there will be duplication of obstacles across groups. I know the group leaders will use their discretion, that previously stated obstacles do not go unmentioned, for it may well be that they were mentioned for different reasons. While we may have some repetition, I think the group leaders will be able to indicate differences and similarities.

Christman: There are duplications, but obstacles are often viewed in a different context. The first obstacle we examined is probably the easiest to overcome by the profession and by the other hospital workers. It doesn't require more work, more studies, more money. It's a slight shift of attitude. That should be easy to accomplish. Change our lifestyle!

Public Law 1199, the labor issue, was the second obstacle. We too talked about aides and LPNs. Our group agreed that the law is spotty. It depends on the neighborhood in which the hospital is located, its immediate geographic surroundings, and whether it is or is not governmentally affiliated. Tenure considerations differ depending on whether the job climate is stagnant or highly mobile both within and outside the hospital setting.

The difficulty of adapting to lifestyle change generated considerable discussion. Nursing students are socialized to develop the "wrong set of expectations" or a difficult set of expectations for work than we are now trying to bring about in an ALL-RN staff and in primary care. The role induction process creates many problems for the student. Education and service are disconnected; faculty don't practice; students have no behavioral models of excellence or accountability from their faculty; in the clinical learning arena, students have no models of accountability from the RN staff where team nursing prevails. The total orientation to nursing is deep-rooted and needs transplanting.

Political and organizational skill was another area of discussion. I sensed that some nurses believe there was some sense of powerlessness in organizing the various hospital components. I personally don't see this as a longlasting obstacle; these skills are not that difficult to acquire.

We talked about constraints of startup operations; that is, trying to take on the whole organization versus establishing pilot units. Our group concluded that establishing and debugging pilot units was the best way to overcome organizational sluggishness.

Another area under which various topics of discussion could be grouped was lack of leadership. Not only must the lifestyle of staff nurses and middle management change, so it must change for nurse managers and others to fully implement the necessary organizational designs. The careers of many have been secured by maintaining the status quo, and even those who support change must work against their own longstanding attitudes which regard normality as the status quo.

Brown: I would like to express special thanks to my group which was just so great that I'm not sure as a leader whether I was being followed or chased. We began by selecting the nominal group process technique as a methodology for defining the barriers to implementing the ALL-RN staff. Only some of us had experience using it, but it seemed worth a try. The outcome was sixty-one barriers to implementation and obviously here the process was halted in an attempt to categorize all these uncovered barriers. We arrived at ten major categories and I'll try to share those below as expressed by the group.

(1) Supply of RNs. Included in this category were recruitment; maldistribution of nurses; problem of RN resistance to night work; geographical availability of RNs; part-time versus full-time status of RNs; and a high attrition rate for RNs versus a low attrition rate for LPNs or ancillary personnel.

(2) Change in the registered nurse role. This category included the change in role identification; knowledge and skill level of the RN; lack of autonomy—there was considerable discussion about what lack of autonomy really meant, and how it could be expressed in behavioral terms. The discussion resulted in a definition that included clinical knowledge and the competency to use it leading to good decision making and independence in the collegial relationship.

Also under the category of change in the RN role was the peer relationship between the RN, the LPN, and other non RN staff. Others were the questionable ability of the existing nurses to adapt to the new system; the reluctance of staff RNs to accept responsibility or accountability; the poor attitude of some RNs toward performing patient-care tasks; the RN failing to recognize the need for an ALL-RN staff; traditional allegiance to the hospital rather than the patient; failure to uniformly define nursing; conflict between the educational system and nursing practice; redefining of the support systems for nursing; and waste of RN talent. Examples of the latter were rendered in such areas as "with an ALL-RN staff, do we exclude the OR Tech, the ER Tech, the OB Tech, or other such categories, and if we exclude these, would we be inappropriately using RNs?"

(3) Change in organizational structure to enhance professional practice. Changing the documentation or charting methods in the present system was one structural change to facilitate practice. Other changes include organizational restructuring both within and outside nursing service; subjective loyalties to long-term employees; utilization of personnel in nursing management positions; division of labor. The latter point refers to longstanding belief regarding efficiency that forces health-care workers to revert to a functional mode, assuming it most efficient. This division of labor creates a barrier to the professional accountability of the ALL-RN staff. Finally, the effects on other departments of change in organizational structure and appropriate salary scales for increased responsibility must be addressed.

(4) Change in standards of practice. In this category we cited proper utilization of levels of RNs and redefining standards or the support systems for nursing. More clearly defined standards of practice would facilitate the restructuring of the organization and so was included in the previous category as well. Clarifying the acuity index or indicators in patient categories for the lay public was another item and finally methods for measuring RN care versus mixed staffing.

(5) Outside considerations. Here we considered tenure and non profes-

sionals in civil service settings; dealings with labor unions; negative community reactions. As for example, if many nursing assistants and LPNs live in the
community, a change to an ALL-RN staff would mean loss of jobs for
community residents, which could cause problems in the community.

Another area of concern is the reimbursement of hospital systems by state
rate reviews. The quality of care cannot be an issue in the rate setting
mechanisms now on the books in six states.

Other concerns are licensure laws (the exams are not all the same), political
constraints, and lack of success by previous ALL-RN systems.

(6) Lack of change agent leaders. This category contains one of our longest
listings. I'll try to relay all the shortcomings we have as leaders: lack of nurse
administrators as strategy planners to convince administrators; dealing with
the effect of change on other departments; opposition by the governing
board; the need for education to implement changes; the assurance of positive
input to change within and among departments; overcoming weaknesses and
failures in effecting change without abandoning goals; the tendency for a
leader or change agent to jump on the bandwagon without looking at modifi-
Non-RN personnel don't want to join the staff if they think they are going to
long-range planning for change.

(7) Public relations politics. This category included strong negative reaction in the community; elimination of LPNs already on board; lack of non
RNs when the commitment to an ALL-RN staff is announced to the public (if
you announce the change to an ALL-RN staff too soon, you have difficulty
hiring other staff to keep the system running while you're changing direction.
Non RN personnel don't want to join the staff if they think they are going to
eventually be laid-off); political constraints, subjective loyalties to long-term
employees, and loss of community identity.

(8) Collegial relationship. Obstacles in this category include security and
comfort with the present nurse/physician relationship; nurse reward systems
that emphasize the physician rather than the nurse or patient; territoriality on
the part of physicians' collegial relationships with other departments; power
struggles deriving from increased numbers of RNs compared to lack of
growth in other professional departments; physician acceptance of the registered nurse as colleague.

(9) Physical environment. Discussion centered around variations in the
physical environment. For example, if a progressive care patient moves
through four units in eight days, how can one RN be held accountable or
given a very small unit and an ALL-RN staff, how can staffing be handled
when two RNs at night are too much and one is not enough?

(10) Budget and staffing. This category included such things as cost and
time of data collection and analysis of cost effectiveness and criteria needed
for ALL-RN staffing. Probably the most significant barrier to our discussion
was our awareness at the close of our listing of barriers that we weren't all
talking the same language. Does an ALL-RN staff mean primary nursing and

does primary nursing mean you must have an ALL-RN staff? This is a point that our group would like to explore further with the entire audience.

Carlson: It's not surprising that a group such as this, meeting to discuss an ALL-RN staffing pattern, would arrive at very similar outlines of obstacles. I think our group's approach was a little different and I would like to provide some detail regarding it.

We began with the outside constraints. One such constraint was the outside accrediting bodies, that is, the JCAH. The accrediting body sets standards by specifying what is needed to be accredited. If the accrediting bodies do not set a particular standard, there is no incentive to establish it. For those unaware, there is a new standards draft currently out for review. As fantastically advanced as these new standards are under the heading of nursing service, still nowhere is direct patient care by the RN addressed. Registered nurses are still planning, evaluating, directing, supervising. We must supply our input to the nurses developing the new standards.

Some of the state codes posed another outside constraint. These codes reward adherence to the status quo. If you attempt something more creative and fail to, for instance, specify long-term and short-term goals, you will be cited for not conforming and you will not be rewarded for innovation because it's not part of the standards. Innovation is above the standards; it's not even recognized. While accreditation may be advantageous for those who don't meet minimum standards, it is a hindrance for those who perform above such standards. No credit is awarded for performance above the minimum level; in fact, you are cited for failing to carry out certain requirements that the accrediting bodies judge to be important but that you consider unimportant. Our nurse practice acts, even our new act in New York State, still admonish us not to deviate "from the professional or medical regimen." That doesn't promote autonomy and responsibility. If we equate an ALL-RN nursing staff with professional nursing, our nurse practice acts do not offer us professional nursing status. We are still subjected to supervision by doctors, dentists, chiropractors, and osteopaths. That I think is a tremendous obstacle.

I do not view nursing education as being that terrible and the curricula are subject to change. Educators are emphasizing the nursing process. Yet there is a covert problem. Many of the present instructors, like most of us here, came through the diploma school programs. No matter how you do it, you can go on for your BS, your Master's, and ten PhD's, but lingering in our memory and talked about with pride are those three years and having lived through them. Despite the fact that you teach process and autonomy in the baccalaureate program, clinical practice is still done a la the old diploma school days on the unit. Can we change that? I was reminded of the book *Coma*. The female intern or medical student joins a unit with freedom to function, do physical assessments and see patients. In contrast, the female nursing student joins a unit completely restrained, constrained, and that is one of her problems.

Moving from the outside to inside constraints, there are the administrators and the myth of cost effectiveness. Also mentioned, of course, was the nurse/doctor game; trying to get on progress notes and act in a professional manner. That is a problem. We discussed unions, supporting services, lack of unit service management. As we discussed the latter, I was reminded of Luther Christman's article in the *Saturday Review* written in the early 1960s. It was called, "Can a Stewardess Help."

The most significant constraint was mentioned very quickly by Luther Christman. He said you overcome it quickly, just change attitude. Well, Luther, you know I hate to bring up the male/female role. We could take hours going through that particular role because the doctor/nurse game really isn't what it appears to be. It's the male/female game that is being played. All the things you mentioned—the powerlessness, the power, can nursing shed bureaucracy—these are all the constraints. If the staff does not have power to be autonomous because we nurses don't give it to them, then we may have a problem. If we can solve that attitude, Luther, we probably can take care of all the other constraints without any problem whatsoever.

Werner: We were fortunate in having many nursing service administrators, a healthy number of inservice educators, two mid-level administrator supervisors, two head nurses, and two members of national organizations in our group. So we had a wide range of contributions as far as value systems and priorities were concerned. Using a brainstorming technique, we saw as obstacles to implementing an ALL-RN staff a number of things which when I began to put them together last night fell into natural groupings.

The first obstacle we noted was the traditional structure of nursing as a discipline. That is, a discipline viewed as a service department rather than a clinical specialty, requiring employees who perform the tasks of a service department rather than clinical practitioners who care for patients and are accountable for the outcomes of their practice. If we saw it that way, we wouldn't be able to have anything but RNs, would we? Nursing seen in the world in which we all live is a bundle of tasks rather than a sequential process.

The next obstacle was the value system of nursing leadership and the nursing staff. We must bring these two together because in some cases they are diametrically opposed to each other. Our group felt that perhaps it was important to us to maintain the status quo rather than to risk the unknown— a much more comfortable position. Perhaps it is more important to protect the nonprofessional's job security than promote competent care of patients. That's our dilemma. We are unwilling to betray our friends and assistants, people who have been so loyal to us, LPNs and nursing assistants, in order to promote an elite system. When said that way, we are being put in a position of doing someone in to gain something that is precious to our profession. Within our own value system it looks as though "We are going to get what we want at the price of someone else's security." We did not enter this profession because we were more concerned about ourselves than others and it's very difficult for us now to take a hard look at the facts, but that is our dilemma.

We saw resistance on the part of staff nurses to:
(1) Assume the inherent accountability for outcome of practice.
(2) Follow the progressive care of the patient, be it at his bedside, in the sitz bath, or on the hospital lawn.
(3) Become involved in and attentive to a patient's crisis or the agony of his chronicity.
(4) To develop a significant relationship with the patient's family.

As I listened to Sylvia talk about the old world in which so many of us were brought up, I recalled that we were not permitted to become involved with patients or their families; it was unprofessional. Sylvia Carlson and I come out of a school one year apart. We never wore nametags, lest someone discover that we were persons. We were blue and white striped bundles of competence. I don't know, Sylvia; we've changed. Our professionalism was measured by the length of our hair from our collar and our skirt from the floor, and it is very hard to change our heads. There is a great resistance in our profession to risking the collegial relationship with the patient's physician. If we have an ALL-RN staff, the relationship centers around the patient and not the doctor's orders.

There is a great difficulty with the value system espoused in the educational component of nursing. The emphasis is on the clerical component of nursing where the RNs are care planners and care organizers rather than care givers. Unless we alter our world view and provide behavioral models for students, we will perpetuate this system. We have got to turn this world around so that students can have role models they can aspire to, and they have got to see that in their faculty.

We see a real fear in provoking labor unrest resulting in the unionization of either professional nurses or the auxiliary staff. We are concerned about the image of the professional association, the ANA, as a labor union, as presented by the Commission on Economic and General Welfare. We see a dilemma presented by the prospect of the Bachelor's Degree as a requirement for the entry into practice, coupled by an increase in schools for nonprofessionals.

There is a great fear, and it's a myth, that an ALL-RN staff will be too costly. It is perceived as a Cadillac model. Those of us who have data know that this is a myth. One obstacle is an accounting system in some hospitals that obscures the real nursing costs and propagates an image of excessive spending with boards, administrators, and certainly physicians. If you are looking at cost effectiveness in health care, this could be a problem.

We are worried about an RN labor market that won't respond to the demand. Wouldn't it be terrible if we said we were going to have an ALL-RN staff and then couldn't fill the positions?

We see some professional deficiencies in nursing as real obstacles to implementing an ALL-RN staff: inadequate behavioral models; ignorance of nursing administration and the nursing staff in negotiation and in implementing change; an unwillingness to risk an uncertain future; inexperience in the political area, both within our own hospitals and in the outside world, which inhibits our influence; uncertainty about the consequences of a system in which the care givers, an ALL-RN staff, are bright, probably young, autonomous professionals, while the leadership group, the administrators and supervisors, are not clinically competent and base their authority on the status of the position; medical staff resistance, which is extremely subtle but powerful. The threat, the implications of a competent nursing staff, implies a great deal of power. Physicians are practicing in a climate of mistrust. They are all too well aware of the women's movement. They are all too well aware, even now, of nurses who are more and more competent, more and more knowledgable. It's a great threat, but it's not only a personal threat, it's a concern about the power base in our institutions.

We raised some questions that we hope will be discussed by this group. We are concerned about the implication of an ALL-RN staff that might not be clinically competent. What would happen if we had an ALL-RN staff and everyone was not clinically competent, particularly the leadership group? It occurred to us that we could build an ALL-RN staff composed essentially of part-timers or of agency nurses. Would we be willing to settle for such a group?

Alfano: I'm going to use the moderator's prerogative and answer one question. I don't know what would happen if we had an ALL-RN staff of incompetent RNs. I just want to know what we're doing now with mixed staffs who are incompetent.

McClure: Like the other group leaders, I was impressed with the quality of discussion in our group. I'm not certain that leadership was needed; it evolved from the group.

We also discussed the availability of RNs—a grave concern for most of us. Many questioned whether the supply of RNs can accommodate the personnel demands of an ALL-RN staff. And geographic mal-distribution is a serious problem. We were, however, heartened by Barbara Brown's presentation which reassured us that even in critical situations changes can occur. The discussion then moved to salary levels. One member works in an area where ALL-RN staffing has been tried, but the salary level is not competitive. It is actually lower for nurses joining an ALL-RN staff. We must offer, at the least, competitive salaries, if not better salaries, to successfully develop a model to which nurses will respond.

Lack of effective leadership was a constraint noted time and again during our discussion. Many of us have witnessed ineffective leaders at high levels of administration. June Werner's comment about our lack of expertise in the political arena is very serious, particularly in our own agencies. Allowing the medical staff and administration to lead us is certainly not constructive. We must develop more effective, strong, visible nursing leaders who in turn will recruit and properly utilize strong middle-level managers. That point was emphasized on several occasions.

Lack of nursing leadership in ANA is another problem. The E&GW Program led many directors of nursing to leave the ANA and that raises questions about the future of professional standards. A group member from Virginia informed us that they have formed a separate organization for E&GW, which has not thrilled the ANA. It might be worth further investigation for those of us interested in the problem. Lack of administrative effectiveness cannot be overlooked. Historically, nursing administration has not been viewed in a very important light. In fact, the nursing profession seems to think that administrative responsibilities should be relegated to the least able. Clinical preparation has been the order of the day and preparation in administration has been denigrated. Apologies were in order if you chose to pursue nursing administration. Now we're suffering the consequences. We must begin to see ourselves as one of the specialties of the profession.

An interesting point made during this discussion was that nursing leaders should begin to view themselves as business women, particularly directors of nursing. They should learn to use economic terms effectively and train middle managers and some staff members to think and speak similarly.

Tied to this issue is the lack of education for nursing service administration. For some time now good programs have been few in number and certainly poorly distributed geographically. Three doctoral programs for nursing service administration that were recently established are having difficulty recruiting faculty because so few people in nursing administration have doctorates. This chicken and egg problem is not readily resolved. Perhaps the best preparation in nursing service administration is a degree in that specialty area, but coursework in other fields such as business and political science is meaningful for directors of nursing.

We then talked about all aspects of our profession by role conflicts as described by Barbara Brown. Most poignant are the efforts of a female profession to maintain individuals as professionals who are also wives and mothers and the problems of absenteeism and turnover created by this conflict. We discussed day care, for example, as one means to ease conflict of this nature. A nurse recruiter in the group informed us that day care centers are on the decline in hospitals, which I can well understand. When I worked in a hospital in Philadelphia, we considered establishing a day care center but found that our night nurses saw it as a way to avoid night duty, and we promptly decided we would not open a day-care center. Keeping a night staff is essential. In any case, we talked about the fact that evenings and nights are bigger problems than days, yet we speak of DAY-care centers.

Another aspect of this role conflict problem is that women tend to follow men geographically. So many constraints are placed on women who attempt to work and maintain a profession; often these women over compensate by trying to do more in both roles than most people do in one. The traditional role of the female continues to create problems both at home and at work. For example, at home one expects that a sick child will be cared for by the mother even though both parents work. One group member does share this responsibility with her husband; they take turns staying home with their sick child, but I think they are a rare couple. In the work setting, there are certain expectations about female behavior. We believe that a fair number of women are still buffaloed by male administrators, male physicians, and other male colleagues, especially in power struggles.

We too discussed the negative reaction of unions as a constraint to change. I do agree that it is possible to transfer people from dead-end jobs to better career opportunities in other departments. But this is very difficult for a union to buy in such settings as New York City, for example. The diminishing supply of union jobs aggravates their concern. Other areas besides New York City are closing beds and hospitals. No matter how you look at this issue, it does, in fact, decrease the number of union jobs available in an already tight market.

We also talked about the problem of an ALL-RN staff, if the RNs are organized in collective bargaining units and strike. Areas that have had RN strikes have reportedly soured administrators toward ALL-RN staffs. However, with an ALL-RN staff the registered nurses may be less likely or less motivated to strike, recognizing that they are the only individuals responsible for care of the patients. With a mixed staff, one group goes out and the other shoulders the burden. Perhaps the nurse in an ALL-RN staff would impose greater constraints on herself to vote to strike.

We discussed many of the same issues as other groups—the attitudes of the staff and socialization into traditional roles, task orientation, direct care measures relegated to aides and considered inappropriate for the professional nurse. Many attitudinal changes must take place if we intend to achieve a level of professional nursing. There is a lack of professional identity and a blue-collar attitude toward the job of nursing—where the high point of the day is clocking out and the emphasis is on the amount of money earned. It is a notion that nursing is more a job than a professional commitment. Related to this is the problem of older staff members with the clip boards and how to deal with people in supervisory positions who have been around so long that it is difficult to let them go, but who are not close enough to retirement to be eased out of their position. That's a real problem for many of us.

Insitutions attempting to modify primary nursing are a potential problem. Modified primary nursing very often only destroys the whole concept of accountability. Such hybrid approaches could damage primary nursing beyond recognition. The greatest fear is that primary nursing would be identified with these approaches and would share in their failures.

Like others, we talked about the problem of night staffing and weekend staffing. We were particularly concerned about primary nursing on weekends that are very low in staff support. Some members of our group had union contracts that called for every other weekend off. Operating with 50 percent of staff two days out of the week can create serious problems. One group member did emphasize the importance of examining the weekend workload and realistically assessing staffing needs.

We also discussed decentralization as it related to nurses reporting to medical directors rather than the director of nursing. In some parts of the country an assistant director in charge of surgical nursing does not report to the director of nursing in a line relationship, but reports to the director of surgery, a physician, a surgeon. This creates problems in raising standards because it undermines the influence of the director of nursing. Also, in some hospitals certain departments such as the operating room or the out-patient department do not report to the director of nursing, making implementation of a total plan very difficult. We concluded our discussion with the entry into practice problem. An ALL-RN staff is not comprised of a particular type of nurse with a particular set of characteristics but rather many types of nurses some of whom are better or less prepared for the job at hand. In relation to this, LPNs are earning sufficient salaries now and with fringe benefits added, their cost effectiveness warrants close examination. The literature supports the decline in use of the LPN, and one contributing factor is the close proximity of their salary range to that of the RN.

Our discussion ended with the lack of opportunities for associate degree and diploma nurses to obtain the baccalaureate degree. The difficulty stems not only from educational preparation but also from the bitterness many experience. This bitterness has led many associate degree and diploma nurses to fight against some of the proposals that we have initiated dealing with delivery of professional care through ALL-RN staffing and primary nursing.

Donaho: It is interesting to observe the diverse categorization of similar issues across the different discussion groups. I would like to make some generalizations before reporting the group discussion. The first generalization is that generalizations are dangerous to make. As we identified all of those issues presenting a challenge—a slightly more positive word than obstacle—it became apparent that matters were perceived as issues in some settings and not in others. So, to state that everything identified was an issue to be dealt with in all settings is foolhardy. As nurse leaders, we must assess our own situations, determine the direction we wish to take, and plan our strategies for achieving those goals. Secondly, it bears stating that the change process takes time and must proceed with patience toward our goals.

We literally brainstormed for one and a half hours identifying the challenges. We arrived at roughly thirty-seven of them. We were sidetracked now and again thinking we should discuss certain issues rather than continue brainstorming without interruption. Then, we began to focus on some issues to try to order them in a meaningful way.

Interestingly enough, one of the first challenges that we identified was inadequate knowledge of the nursing process itself. That indeed is an obstacle if you are planning to establish a program to implement the nursing process. If you do not know what it is, you cannot do it. Considering that the nursing process in itself may be a deterrent, we went on to identify why.

(1) Implementing the nursing process forces the staff to identify cause and effect relationships. In some instances this is a new experience and may not be a very comfortable one.

(2) The nursing process is not understood, not only by RNs, but by the medical profession, administrators, and other disciplines with which nursing interacts. That ignorance becomes a deterrent to learning about the profession which may appear as a threat.

(3) To implement change, the staff must abandon its task orientation, with which it may be very comfortable.

(4) There are varying degrees of willingness to assume accountability for the nursing process.

(5) A negative attitude toward the system exists within the profession. What is the value in delivering care? I've even heard a staff wonder aloud whether it can stand a particular patient for the length of his or her stay in the hospital. These value judgments and attitudes must be reconciled if an ALL-RN staff and primary care are instituted.

(6) Evaluation based not on the adherence to the nursing process. We still tend to evaluate performance on attendance, appearance, and other peripheral issues, rather than on effective use of the nursing process.

To summarize, we must begin to connect the links in the nursing process to accountability and preparation of the provider. By this, I refer not only to entry-level education into the profession, but also to keeping abreast of developments in the field and changes in professional standards.

We then turned to the heading that we chose to label perceptions of nursing and nurses by others.

(1) Nursing is perceived by others as nonessential. There are ORTs, nursing assistants, clericals, LPNs—a huge listing of titles that we've created within the nursing hierarchy.

(2) The perception of the non-nursing staffs that nurses aren't doing nursing anyway. So why are they needed?

(3) The perception that nursing has always performed certain tasks, albeit

of a non-nursing nature such as lab work, housekeeping, or transporting. Why not continue the system the way it is?

(4) One new health-care intervention can be utilized in both a positive and a negative way. That is, systems engineering studies have validated time needed to perform tasks in nursing. Many of the systems we are using are task oriented which defeat implementation of the nursing process. I'm not disputing these studies in terms of the patient classification systems on which staffing is built. But while these systems continue on a task-oriented basis, we are creating another quagmire.

(5) The medical staff's perception of and complacency with their role as captain of the ship. That perception lingers regardless of how it's defined.

Another category that we selected was nurses' contribution to others perceptions of us.

(1) Reality of nursing practice. Nurses are willing to relegate, delegate, or disregard. Without a system that accommodates neglect, the staff is accountable and this may be an uncomfortable position.

(2) Paucity of our own studies and research reports that define and support the nursing process, its purpose, and how it can be accomplished.

(3) Absence of a clear definition of nursing built on a value system that we can support as individuals and as a profession.

(4) Breaches in nursing, whether between the staff and administration or between nurses, through which we fail to support one another. Our conflicts often focus on personalities rather than issues. We do not know how to disagree and confront others while averting personal feuds, and I think this failing is a major deterrent for us as a profession.

(5) Our rigidity and unwillingness to reorganize or change. We tried to recount all the reasons why we can't do something. We tend toward a negative approach rather than one in which we can identify our preferences and ascertain how to achieve our goals. Our colleagues tire of asking nurses to do something and getting myriad reasons why it cannot be done.

Absence of actions that reinforce a value system was our next category. Under this heading we noted:

(1) Our tendency to stroke the negative. We ensure that mistakes are well documented, but the staff seldom hears what was done well. We must find ways to increase positive feedback.

(2) Lack of nursing representation on joint medical staff committees. The term itself irritates me since representatives come from pharmacy, therapeutics, and utilization review. But still I think across the country articulate nursing representation on these committees is lacking. Collegial relationship are not fostered by absenteeism at the committee table.

(3) The evaluation processes that are task-oriented and not related to implementation of the nursing process. This issue was mentioned before but is appropriate here as well and bears repeating.

Labor relations was the next category and this has already been fully addressed in terms of the power of unions and the focus on members relating not to the delivery system but to protection of the membership. At times we run the risk that some matters involving unions will be linked with discrimination, whether intended or not. Also under this broad heading was the perceptions of order and level of jobs in a hospital organization. Nursing assistants are perceived in a better light than housekeeping or laundry staff even though all may be on the same pay scale. So at a time when we might like to make a lateral move, we find that the image we have created prohibits such a move, since over time we've supported the implication that individuals in nursing are better than in housekeeping or dietary. We now must live with and deal with that perception of level and order in a hierarchy because we've built it for a long time.

Under separate heading we dealt briefly with some of the legislation on the federal, state, and local levels, and the rate review processes. Again, I emphasize that these challenges that we identified have both pluses and minuses. They may be opportunities as well as obstacles. We are not alone in our concerns regarding the rate review process, the constraints of cost containment, responses to the consumer, and consumer encroachment into the realm of decisions we feel are our prerogative and territorial right; this is one of the principal paranoias of medicine, but it's going to rapidly creep into nursing if we don't begin to address the issue. The willingness to reimburse some third-party payers for some levels of care sets constraints on our profession, forcing us to make the best possible use of personnel. We need documentation to support utilization and the value levels we place on units of service.

Our discussion moved to the issue of the change process itself, which presents a challenge and possibly a deterrent. One of the first aspects of this issue that we identified was fear of the unknown and the inertia it propagates. Where in the world do you start to make a change of this magnitude and how do you control it? There is resistance to change deriving from both fear of failure and fear of success. There are some people who have an equal amount of fear in both directions. Not understanding the rationale for change is certainly an obstacle to implementing it. When change proceeds with any rapidity, many people are unable to accept it simply because of its speed, the expectation of taking on the changes at a rate that cannot be dealt with. If change is not understood, it meets resistance. Time for education is required in the process of change. It is an expense, but necessary; if you miss that step, change will not occur as hoped or planned.

For lack of a better heading under which to group other issues, we chose as our label characteristics of nurses.

(1) Role identification. What is nursing, what is not nursing? Personnel will covet the duties they enjoy whether these are nursing duties per se. We must allow time to focus on role identification because nurses have assimilated it, it is part of their way of doing things, and they're not going to drop it just because you and I or the head nurse says they should. Passive resistance

among the staff exists as a result of this role issue. If you doubt that, initiate a policy then monitor it and see how it is implemented.

(2) Unit interdependence has been identified and referred to. It speaks to the issue of loyalty whether real or imagined within a group, whether related to elimination of jobs or what have you. We have spent years creating that interdependence which we've called team nursing. We've spent years ensuring that some tasks are delegated, that certain personnel are used, that nurses become dependent upon them. Suddenly, we're saying that isn't the way it is. Why don't you catch up with us and get back on the right track. You don't undo things as quickly as that; and if you recall how long we have been working to get team nursing under way in this country, it's going to take probably that long if not longer to undo what we have done.

(3) Nurses are unaccustomed to nurse-to-nurse support. We fend for ourselves because we are convinced that it is inappropriate to solicit support. We never make mistakes or at least we never admit to erring. Consequently, support for the mistakes of others is not a familiar or comfortable experience for us. Yet it's part of our definition of the nursing process—to be supportive of patients and families. But we don't always translate that to support of ourselves and employ the techniques that are part of our trade.

(4) Complacency regarding current status and care levels within our profession. This doesn't entirely translate to our behavior however. We're a group of health-care providers that wear different hats. When we're working, we know we are providers; when we're at home we are part of the consumer group and very willing to criticize. That's when we know we're not satisfied with what we're doing. However, in our own unit trying to maintain stability, we indicate that we are satisfied with the status quo and we really don't want change.

Certain isolated issues are applicable and yet are difficult to categorize. These are availability and turnover, the professional entry system, our ability to handle conflict, the availability of support systems necessary in care delivery and our efforts to move the non-nursing staff into those support systems. Just dealing with emotions. Many of these issues are emotionally charged; they become irrational and once people begin to deal with irrational issues, you never get back to the rational ones. You might as well call the meeting to a halt. Then we also concluded that our own management style can either be a challenge, a deterrent, or an asset, and we need to look at that. As we talked about many of these issues, someone in the group said, "You know, we continue to be our own worst enemy."

Alfano: That was an excellent summary of the issues and obstacles and challenges that the group as a whole has pointed out. Some of us never did ascribe to either team nursing or functional assignment at any point in time in terms of the delivery of nursing services. We have less trouble reaccommodating change and are not plagued with the system.

My group covered most of the issues identified by previous speakers. Rather than repeat these issues, I will look at the process of nursing. The group wanted to consider strategies as they related to specific obstacles. We felt that if we were going to define or identify obstacles to implementing an ALL-RN staff, it might be interesting to also identify ways of coping with the process of change to make it more feasible.

Nursing service and nursing education must take a hard look at services required of the nursing profession. Doing so will inevitably raise such questions as what does nursing wish to do as a profession, what is its stance, what does it choose to deliver as a service, and what is the preparation necessary to deliver that service. Having addressed these issues, we then consider the delivery system that will best support the role of the nurse. Beyond that, we must arrive at a philosophy of nursing care, and a level of competence at which it must be practiced. We are then in a position to determine the nature of preparation necessary to practice at the chosen level, rather than reviewing the obstacles to practice at a level below that at which we should be practicing.

I would like to open discussion on two major challenges noted. Are primary nursing and an ALL-RN staff necessarily mutually inclusive? Must you have an ALL-RN staff for primary nursing or must you do primary nursing with an ALL-RN staff? The other issue is what happens with an ALL-RN staff if RNs are incompetent; how do we cope with that? Maybe the hidden question is whether RNs are really competent to deliver nursing care? This is a question in the minds of many, especially LPNs. I would like to ask Luther Christman if he would care to respond to some issues raised here.

Christman: I get concerned when sexism is brought out as an issue because I think it's too seductive and an easy cop-out. I hope that nursing doesn't assume the position of defending lack of progress on the grounds that this is a sexist world. No matter who is in the power arrangement, those in control don't wish to share their power with those who have none. That's why we had student revolts on campus, black/white confrontation, latino/white confrontation, and male/female confrontation. Then there are subgroups within those groups who don't want to share power. I think there is a great reluctance on the part of women in nursing to share power with men in nursing and it's very obvious. Ask any of the men, they'll tell you. We speak from the lowest, we're the smallest minority in the whole profession, two percent. I view the profession as a minority member, and I see this portrayal of power all the time. Just let me raise some questions to get at this issue. What literature is more sexist than the nursing literature? All nurses are female. I have had the word he/she deleted from all the articles that I have written by every editor of every nursing journal in the United States to be replaced by she. I know that women in other groups absolutely insist that sexist pronouns be eliminated but don't hear any nurses rising to correct the nursing literature.

All physicians are male. That's ridiculous. With the huge enrollment of women in the medical colleges around the country, "he" doesn't apply to physicians at all. I have yet to see a woman patient. In the literature, all patients are "he." All this misleading, emotional, stressful verbiage, all the time. "All hospital administrators are male." I taught hospital administration on one university campus and there were a fair number of women students in those classes. Yet we allow this absolute stereotyping to cloud our thinking.

Just let me raise a few more questions or comments. Men and women behave more alike when they are nurses. I am concerned about my male colleagues in the profession. They're just as apathetic about advanced education as women. They're just as resistant to change. The stereotypical nurse behavior is uniform across both sexes. It isn't physicians or hospital administrators who are asking nursing to keep education and service separate. No other profession does that and yet has any power. All the powerful professions have united it. They have men and women in those professions but they haven't separated as nurses have. Other professions have one generic means of entry. They're not plagued by in-fighting over who is a professional and how you get professional status. It has nothing to do with male/female.

Consider the universities,—nurses don't want equality on the campus,—if they had it they would be required to earn the same credentials as the rest of the faculties, both men and women in all other professions. Nurses have shown an enormous reluctance to becoming fully credentialed and, as such, holding equal power arrangements with the rest of the university faculties. That has nothing to do with male/female, because many of the male nurses who have university faculty appointments refuse to get doctorates, as do female nurses. It's a nurse problem not a male/female problem.

A series of stereotypes cloud clear thinking about the issues. I have never heard any nurses in our hospital talk about men keeping them back, whether physicians or hospital administrators or male nurses. I have heard the reverse, there is admiration for these women by physicians, hospital administrators, and scientists. It isn't the outside world that keeps nurses from organizing politically effective organizations; nurses are divided or apathetic. They never unite in powerful lobbying efforts (in Washington or the state capitals) to advance their ideas or to get nurse appointments to powerful positions, task forces, or committees. If they do, it's tokenism. We either react with apathy and withdraw or we become overly aggressive and so hostile that we are blinded to the problems. I'm suggesting that we should view this issue for what it is. Power and power sharing do not arrive overnight; they come when one gains skill in dealing with the people who have the power.

Alfano: Thank you, Luther. It was important to clarify that issue and to recognize that it has nothing to do with the existence of an ALL-RN staff. Sometimes we do tilt at windmills. I think, Luther, that you would give credence to the fact that nursing, because it is a predominantly female profession, is as a result underpaid and lower in status.

Christman: That is true of some male-dominated professions. Clergy do as poorly or worse than nurses, and they are predominantly male. It's the thing that society does to people. I'm not saying that it is right.

Audience: I do not presume to argue with Luther Christman so I will direct a question to the group. How many of you here have a woman as your chief executive officer or your hospital administrator? Raise your hands. One, two, three, four, five. Of those hospital administrators and chief executive officers who are women, how many are nuns? (Four hands raised.)

Werner: This issue will not go away. I've been 5 feet tall all my adult life. It's been a problem. It's the same as being a woman. I don't think we should focus our emotional energies on this. There is nothing we can do about it. We are what we are. For those of us in administrative jobs, it could be a problem. Is your salary commensurate with your educational preparation and your experience like others, because they tend to be men. If you are in nursing service administration, one part of your world is comprised of women and then you go down the hall to the luncheon meeting and you are the only one. It can make you a little schizophrenic. You are in the minority. If we focus on this, as we have for a long time in this profession, we don't have enough energy to focus on matters within our control. If we just focused all our energies on accountability for the clinical profession and became so successful at providing nursing care in our institution, we would be indispensable. Now, I think indispensibility is a quality that will give us a lot more power than being male or female. I think nursing can be indispensable to the whole health-care system in this country. That's where we need to put our energies.

Donaho: We must begin to focus on the issues at hand and develop effective strategies to deal with those issues. We cannot afford to cloud matters with personal confrontations, whether between ourselves as professional nurses or with the hospital administrator or the physician. If we attack on personal fronts we should not deserve to be in that leadership position and we will never be indispensable; if we keep to the issues at hand, to participate in the delivery of health care and provide distinctive nursing care, then we will be indispensable and not until then.

Alfano: On that particular note, let us address the question of whether primary care implies an ALL-RN staff or an ALL-RN staff implies primary care. Would anyone care to start us off on that issue?

Burt: I suggest that we turn the question to our audience. We have quite a few primary nurses here. I would like them to get involved in this question again.

Audience: I would like someone to tell me what they mean when they say primary nursing. I've talked to many people who say they do primary nursing, and everyone defines it differently. My concern is that each of us sitting here has our own idea or definition that differs from what Marie Manthey described primary nursing to be. I think we should clarify that.

Alfano: Of course one answer is that since Marie Manthey coined the term, primary nursing must be as she defined it and anyone who uses her term has misused the system because the person who generates the term has first claim to its definition.

Audience: Well, I think that's the problem that we're experiencing in the nursing community. People have modified the term. As Doctor McClure said, "the modification of primary nursing is destroying it." I think we need to address the issue. If we are not doing primary nursing as defined by Manthey, why do we call it primary nursing?

Alfano: The only answer is that those who are doing primary nursing, or who call what they are doing primary nursing, had better define what they say they are doing.

Audience: I used to use the term primary nursing to define what I did. I will not use the term any longer because what I do is not what I find others defining primary nursing as. What I consider I'm doing is nursing care. The nurse is the care giver. She is the primary person giving care because she is the only person giving care. Obviously this does not agree with the definition of others. I do not feel we need an ALL-RN staff to do what I've heard other people define as primary nursing. I feel we need an ALL-RN staff to do nursing care because the RN is the only one qualified to give that care.

What is nursing care? What is our philosophy of nursing? New graduates of programs today want to be "little doctors"; they are all interested in physical assessment. They are borrowing from medicine. We've given so much away to the nurses aides and the LPNs that nursing has nothing left, so now we do what the doctors do. Which means we are still under the subjugation of doctors rather than doing nursing, where we need no one to supervise us and we can do that on our own.

Audience: I'm in an institution where we are doing primary nursing. We do not have an ALL-RN staff. I would predict that we will end up with this, but I do have our job description which our primary nurses just rewrote, having functioned for one year. I would like to read it to you. "The primary nurse gives comprehensive and individualized patient care from admission to discharge. This is accomplished through assessing, planning, implementing, evaluating, and supervising the care given to the patients assigned to the nurse. The nurse is responsible and accountable for the nursing management and care given to her patients on a twenty-four-hour basis." All our RNs are not primary nurses. Our part-time staff and our nurses who pick up the assignment function as associate nurses do not have twenty-four-hour accountability. Our primary nurses do.

Alfano: Are all of your care givers RNs?

Audience: Yes, our nurses are giving total patient care. This is a rehabilitation facility. There are times in the rehab when what you need is another back and another pair of hands. That is the job of the nursing assistants—to provide that second pair of hands or the back that they need. Otherwise, total patient care is given by the primary nurses. They want to give it.

Alfano: In other words, your nursing assistants give care only with the nurse.

Audience: They are basically assigned functional tasks, such as passing the water pitchers, making the beds, which they may do with the nurse if she has time, but that is their assignment.

Audience: Do you have RNs in your organization who are not primary nurses?
Audience: Yes, we do.
Audience: There are RNs then who are performing task-oriented functions.
Audience: No, but they do not assume the responsibility of the primary nurse. Generally, these are our part-time people and they do not carry primary patients. They are working as associate nurses. They carry the patient load, but they do not have the same accountability as the primary nurse. She has twenty-four-hour, seven day a week accountability.
Audience: Therefore, the part-time RN at a certain hour who needs to know what to do with that patient has access to that primary nurse twenty-four hours a day.
Audience: No, she has access to a well-done care plan and a communications system. With our system I think we have as much continuity of care as you can get. We have the same part-time nurse picking up the same patient assignment every time she comes on duty. We have the same nurses sharing a patient assignment on two shifts. We have rotating positions so when you rotate to another shift, you're carrying the same patient assignment. Now they're carrying six patients, three are their primary patients, three belong to the person on the second shift. We have assumed that we must have primary nursing on two shifts, seven days a week. Our night shift does function differently. They are modeled on a unit nursing system.
Audience: At our institution we do primary nursing. We're using practical nurses out of necessity now as the associate nurse. In other words, the associate nurse relieves the primary nurse on her day off. I take exception to

Marie Manthey's advocacy of LPNs as primary nurses. We find using the LPN as an associate nurse difficult, and I can see the move of phasing out the LPN and bringing in ALL-RNs.

Audience: I take exception to RNs as associate nurses.

Audience: May I just throw one other title in here as long as everybody is confusing definitions? Why don't we toss in modular nursing and see what we do with that? It's up to the individual institution whether you wish to have nurses such as the part-timer or the agency nurse play the role of the primary nurse. I think they feel that the primary nurse is that person who is accountable. My conception of modular nursing is using different levels to deliver care, some being primary nurses which are exclusively RNs augmented by LPNs and aides.

Alfano: In supportive roles. So we now have one more term that we can hide behind.

Werner: We have been working towards primary nursing at Evanston Hospital since 1971. One of the things that's wrong with primary nursing is its title. Terrible title. Sylvia Carlson has a bumper sticker that says, "Let's stamp out primary nursing"; I want to say let's stamp out the title primary nursing. As we see it evolve over the years, primary nursing is a system in which a nurse is accountable for the outcomes of nursing care for her or his patient.

We have elected as a profession to divide our clinical practice into process, basically the four that we all know. Some of us have further divided the components; we have six at Evanston. Yet the primary nurse is accountable for the outcomes of each step of the process and holistically for the outcomes of care for any given patient.

The philosophy we developed at Evanston specified that we would deliver competent, humane, individualized care to each patient and his family, because the illness doesn't happen to the patient alone, it happens to his family. As we proceeded to implement our philosophy, we considered Marie Manthey's model. It would never fit at Evanston because an LPN cannot be used as a primary nurse, particularly because we defined nursing as a process in which one had to be accountable for the outcomes of care. We proceeded with a pilot project on one unit, which I'm willing to admit we set up so that we would succeed, and have proceeded ever since then—started on Valentines Day of 1972, it was such a good omen—and have proceeded. We now have a fully implemented model. It's not perfect, but it's very good, and our patients, their families, and even our physicians feel it's good. While they were changing their mind from it's ridiculous to it's good, a lot of us aged. However, we did not lose our relationship with them. We identified the behavior that we couldn't live with and kept our relationship with them, and now we've got colleagues.

We have moved at Evanston from a staff of 33 percent RNs in 1971 to almost 75 percent now, which means that out of any four care givers, one of them is a nonprofessional. All patients are assigned to RNs. Sometimes an RN has an assistant who is not a professional nurse but could be an LPN or nursing assistant. Now however most of our nursing assistants are student nurses who are on our payroll—terrific recruiting. Yet, we did not focus on what nursing does for patients, but what do patients need and how can we provide it in an incremental way. I would like to think that in ten years we will refine this model with input from our staff and patients because we've learned to listen to patients and families. I tried to eliminate the title primary nursing, and my staff wouldn't hear of it. They wanted to be primary nurses.

Accountability is the key. You won't relegate functions to a nursing assistant for which you are accountable; you'll check, you'll monitor. If you're really committed in a system which rewards you for that kind of behavior, which allows you to bend the policy every now and then because it's good for patients, which gives you professional clout if you're a staff nurse, you won't mind if anybody calls you up at night and says, "Listen, about this patient, I really don't understand, let me tell you what's happening," you won't because you will be acting like a professional. The key is truly the accountability. I don't understand what the young lady means when she says we have primary nursing on days and on nights. If I'm a primary nurse, it doesn't matter when I work. That case load of patients is mine. In that sense it's very much like the medical model.

Christman: I think the whole term is wrong. I have never been happy with it. I suppose it comes out of an earlier experience before primary nursing got in the literature. In 1953, we arranged the care in a hospital in which I was then director of nursing so that there was nurse/physician team management of each individual patient. The physician carried on the usual physician accountability for physician care, but nurses began to pick up in a different way than team nursing which was then running riot. They worked out complementary efforts and planned together. I just wonder if some of the problems and resistance on the part of physician staff isn't over semantics. It takes a while for a physician to realize that the nurse is trying to respond in the "historical physician accountability or physician management" and that all the nurse is trying to do is to become another effective agent for the patient instead of trying to supplant some of the physician effort. I have great question that the strategy of using primary nursing may even be counterproductive.

Alfano: From the standpoint of the National Joint Practice Commission and my visit to the American Medical Association Board of Trustees, nothing seemed to engender more concern and anxiety among the physician group than the term "primary nursing." They maintained that this was certainly not joint practice and feared the concept of patient ownership, which leads to "my" patients, "my" nurse, etc.

If we're talking about language and semantics, I would like to call your attention to two words. One is *case load*. People who carry around loads get very tired. If we are really dealing with people and we are not task oriented, we don't have case loads. The other is *order*; as long as one functions on orders, anybody's orders—nurses, physicians—one is not at liberty to use discretion, to adapt or modify, or to make discriminating judgments; one merely follows the orders. From the standpoint of accountability, if you use registered nurses, it doesn't matter what your delivery system is because I would like to remind you that legally you are accountable regardless of your delivery system. If you use registered nurses, the most fascinating thing is that you may then use any kind of delivery system because by having the most prepared person, you now have options to modify systems which is not true with a mixed staff.

Audience: Luther, I would like to suggest that there is a term that might rile the medical staff more than primary nursing and that's "autonomy."

Christman: That term has been changed to "self-governance" wherever it exists and it only riled certain small elements of the medical staff. The man who asked the question was a member of our staff when the article on autonomous nursing came out, but that title was one given to the authors by the Joint Practice Commission, which was comprised of 50 percent physicians at the time. So, I don't think that any one was trying to defend that term. We no longer talk about autonomy, we talk about self-governance because that's really what it is. No one has autonomy anywhere, no matter which profession, in this day and age, no one has it.

Audience: I think that it is amazing that we're standing here in 1978, talking about an ALL-RN staff. I don't think that any of us would have believed that this would have happened two years ago. My other comment echoes what you just touched upon. The delivery system that one uses is somewhat independent of the type of staff that one has, although using an ALL-RN staff in a functional or a team method of assignment is a waste of the patient's money; and trying to force a nonRN staff into a primary nursing model is an awful lot of wheel spinning. It's not very productive, having worked in both kinds of systems.

Audience: I would just like to comment on primary nursing as it is practiced not just in our hospital but in other Milwaukee hospitals. When the term "primary nursing" is used, it implies that there is a relationship between the nurse and the patient and his family. There is always some relationship when you're working with the patient and a family. Unless that nurse establishes a firm relationship, we do not feel the term "primary" is appropriate even with an ALL-RN staff. In the Milwaukee area when you speak of primary nursing, you are referring to a very solid relationship that continues throughout the patient's hospitalization. If you talk about the ALL-RN staff, I don't know that each nurse can necessarily establish this relationship.

Carlson: Does that mean that a nurse on the other shift who is not assigned a primary patient, who is an associate, may or may not develop a relationship with the patient's family? Is that only the responsibility of the assigned professional?

Audience: All persons regardless of position can establish a relationship.

Carlson: You'll give me that permission if I'm not a primary nurse, if I'm an associate.

Audience: Oh, yes.

Audience: I think the term "primary nursing" is quite confusing. It was confusing to me the first time I heard it, and I immediately asked for a definition of just what it meant. Outside the nursing profession the term could lead to a considerable confusion and hostility, particularly from physicians who might confuse it with primary care. Primary care is one part of a sequence that includes secondary and tertiary care; this is something quite different. We must be much more careful about the terminology that we use.

McClure: You know we in nursing have a lot of trouble with terms. Barbara Donaho and I were discussing our need for labels for almost everything we do. The problem with our labels is that after a time they acquire meaning through their familiarity. Consider the term "nurse practitioner." Until recently, a nurse practitioner was someone who practiced nursing; now we have an entirely new set of expectations for someone that we label nurse practitioner. You and I may refer to all nurses we know as nurse practitioners, but in fact others may think they are something different. It really doesn't matter whether you like the label or whether it even is sensible. If it is accepted, we will use it.

We're stuck with primary nursing at this point. If I advertise for primary nursing positions, it has meaning to people who are now looking for jobs. They arrive with a set of expectations related to what it is they will be doing at my institution. In other words, I think we've dug our own grave here. The term has caught hold, just as nurse practitioner caught hold, and I hate that too.

I would like to make one other comment about primary nursing and an ALL-RN staff. Our experience at my institution has been that if you acquire an ALL-RN staff and you don't do primary nursing, that staff is unrewarded and dissatisfied with the position. Sooner or later you'll lose your staff. I think that primary nursing and an ALL-RN staff go hand in hand if you're interested in job satisfaction for those professional nurses.

Carlson: I agree wholeheartedly. Manthey said herself in a recent AJN article that if you're not doing primary nursing, please don't call it that. She admitted that the term had a sexy, gutsy ring to it that makes people feel it has some substance. I suspect that the nursing community is equating it with the term professional. I think that is the reason for their responses to advertisements for primary nursing. If we began to say we do professional nursing and we will use you in a professional capacity, we may then get people responding to that as well.

This is why I think we must eliminate the term. There are many reasons why it can be confusing; we should replace it with a term that has meaning. We don't call a physician a primary physician; an MD is an MD. Why can't we see for ourselves that an RN is an RN without affixing a qualifying term to the title? We can remove the adjective and say that an RN means something to us in the same way that an MD has significance. It means professional. Then I think we could get rid of the problem. We shouldn't even have registered nurse. We don't say registered doctor or registered lawyer. We just say the term. We insist upon saying registered nurse, we just can't say nurse, and nurse means professional.

Alfano: In other words, if only professional people gave nursing care, we wouldn't have to define it as professional.

Audience: One of the assets of this conference is hearing the different experiences across the country. I appreciated the comment that we should stop generalizing about barriers common to us all because there are none. My experience in Washington suggests that primary nursing is a good term to describe different systems, but it all boils down to delivering the best possible nursing care. Our physicians are willing to try to implement primary nursing, because it means two things to us. First, a patient can say, "my nurse is so and so and there are other people that help give my nursing care, but I have a nurse who will work with me the entire time I'm here, who helps me more than other people in planning what I must do to go home and in working out my problems." Secondly, the nurse follows through as much as possible. When patients transfer to four different units, the primary nurses change out of necessity. But I'm not going to abandon primary nursing in our area.

It bothers me that we will spend so much time talking about the word and not the outcome. It's the same thing with the use of he and she in the literature. You know yourself that when you talk about nurses you find it difficult to stop and say, you know the nurse he/she. Well, let's just forget the language problem and stereotypes will gradually work themselves out of our system. I don't care to point out that I'm a female nurse and I still refer to myself as chairman because I don't want to mess with am I chairperson or chairwoman; it doesn't bother me. I'm the leader of the group and that's that.

I still think we're trying to answer not just the question of how to get to an

ALL-RN staff, but how do we facilitate nurses giving the best nursing they can. I don't care what labels you put on it. I don't care that you have to plan a five year program. It has to do with going back tomorrow to the institution and saying to somebody, not how much work was done but what was the outcome of your work. I don't care whether there's one nurse who is an RN on a unit of forty-five patients, she can pick one patient, she doesn't have to have a case load or a case assignment of six. Try it with one nurse and one patient, and support the effort. We're not 200 barriers, we're 200 possible facilitators if you stop worrying about a program, the PR, the reaction of physicians, just try to practice nursing the way we learned it, which was to assume accountability for "beginning to end" patient care.

Audience: Very hard to follow. I hope I reinforce it because I agree completely. How many remember the slogan "get the emotionalism out of words" and how many remember the original definition of a team leader? It was identity, accountability, and spreading expertise in direct care. Barbara Donaho pointed those out extremely well, we're talking about identity, accountability; we're talking about case assignment instead of task assignment instead of ward assignment. I've approached it from a very different angle. I've said, why are we constantly doing physiological studies without any study framework. Who cares what thirty-four patients temperatures are within one-and-a-half degrees of one another. Who cares what twenty blood pressures are unless you're doing some kind of a physiological study of blood pressures of certain people under certain circumstances, but we have assigned tasks. What bastardized team concepts was exactly the stamping of a label and a system on to a task-oriented assignment organization.

Do you really know how your nursing unit assignments are made? If you don't as an administrator, don't try to make any changes until you find out. Because I can tell you the standards for assignment, the methods of assigning patient care will either make or break change. Now when patients have nurses, the patient has to know the identity, but we have fragmented nurses so, that of course the patient is fragmented. We're trying to eliminate fragmentation of both the practitioner and the patient.

Alfano: I would like to identify what I heard today. I heard that our young nurses do not want to give care because they don't view it as important and our older nurses don't understand the care that has to be given because they are too busy with their clipboards. From those two statements we must conclude that neither the old or young are willing to give care.

We must listen to our inconsistencies and to the way in which both our positives and our negatives become barriers depending upon who is defining them and looking at them. I think it is important to note that all the obstacles, challenges, and barriers that I heard today are barriers, obstacles and challenges that exist in any system where you are trying to deliver anything, and that it really doesn't matter what the staff is. You will still have those obstacles. You will still have union problems; you will still have incompetence; you will still have physician/nurse games; you will still have he/she games; you will still have those in power trying to retain power and those who are not in power trying to get power. It doesn't matter whether these are all RNs, whether they are nonRNs, whether they are practitioners; they are all part of a system that will always be there no matter who you have employed. The real issue here, and it was said very beautifully by the young woman just moments ago, is whether people deserve a certain kind of care. If they deserve that kind of care, then we must find a way to deliver it.

Traditional Intercollegial Relationships

by Barbara J. Brown

Nurse leaders, working toward collegial relationships in a collaborative way, must understand the basic concepts of leadership, power, authority, and influence. These concepts form the basis for discussion of effective persuasion, power, and collaborative relationship techniques.

LEADERSHIP

There are various concepts of leadership that range from the democratic, autocratic, laissez-faire styles to various leadership theories and characteristics. The nurse leader has a responsibility to stimulate her staff by facilitating self-actualization. Individual self-actualization, in accordance with Maslow's hierarchy of need theory, interfaces with organizational needs. Organizational actualization occurs as the cumulative effect of individual actualization satisfying individual needs and complementing organizational needs. This is a synergetic relationship. Effective leadership aids in the assessment of individual needs and their relationship to organizational goals. When individual and organizational needs are simultaneously fulfilled, the highest level of leadership is achieved.

POWER

Dimensions of power will certainly influence collegial relationships. When we consider both power and the concept of leadership that requires nurses to be facilitators of good collegial relationsips, nurses need a very strong self-concept.

We have a responsibility to ourselves for personal growth. We must be effective interactors; we must share energy with others and gain strength from others. When we cooperate and allow equal participation without presumptions of superiority, we are able to share, learn, and grow together. We can pool our knowledge and in doing so garner a strong social power base for nursing.

The social power then becomes interpersonal power, one with the other. Personal power translates to organizational power when each nurse develops a high level of self-esteem and can share knowledge openly without fear of criticism or sanction by others. When staff nurses are given more authority, responsibility, and accountability in the organization of nursing, a system of shared personal power is effected. Such a system is possible with primary nursing.

When personal power is developed, the role change of the nurse is enhanced and facilitated through organizational change.

Formal and functional authority are characteristics of the organization. An individual in a structural organizational position does not necessarily have the personal power characteristics that facilitate organizational power. A director of nursing does not necessarily have power by virtue of the positions in the organization. Use of power requires appropriate use of knowledge in decision-making situations blended with positive verbal and nonverbal communication strategies.

Personal power and positional power are distinctly different dimensions of power and are not necessarily interchangable. For example, some nursing units have leaders no matter what we call them. A staff nurse may provide the nursing personnel with greater motivation toward goal accomplishment than could the head nurse or person who is empowered to lead the group by positional authority. If the leader sets a direction based on organizational goals to which the group objects, it is unlikely that the leader will achieve these goals. Still, that person has by definition an organizational power position.

Fiedler's research on contingency theory[1] includes, as one component, interpersonal relations between the leader and the follower within the framework of the organization. This research considers the follower's acceptance of the leader.

It is considered essential that the follower and the leader have some degree of compatibility. If the leader-nursing administrator creates a climate conducive to professional practice of nursing which is compatible with the nursing staff, then shared power and greater organizational power is initiated. A further development of shared power can be accomplished through a system of staff nurse self-governance similar to medical staffs. Staff nurses should participate in the selection of additional staff members and in the screening of new leaders. If a head nurse leaves a unit, the members of the professional staff should be involved in the selection process that follows. In academe, search and screen committees are always comprised of faculty, and occasionally student, representatives, particularly for committees formed to select leaders at the highest administrative level. A multiple, even interdisciplinary search process is a common approach. How often do hospital administrators or boards of trustees share responsibility with the nursing staff for selection of their new leader when a director of nursing leaves the hospital?

Another component of Fiedler's contingency theory is the nature of the task and the clarity with which it is assigned. For example, the more input by all professional nurses on the staff regarding budget decisions, the less ambiguous the use of time by an individual nurse. Each nurse has a responsibility to maximize time for reasons of cost effectiveness and efficiency. When nurses value themselves and the use of their time in direct patient care and patient care related activities, as in primary nursing, financial accountability becomes shared power.

The third component of Fiedler's contingency theory is the leader's formal authority and actual function in giving rewards and disciplinary actions. This principle could relate to the collective bargaining issue and the strike potential with an ALL-RN staff. Using the self-governance model, each nurse would have organizational power within a structure placing accountability for hiring and firing decisions in the hands of a multiple peer review committee. A staff nurse would share responsibility for credentialing whomever worked as colleagues. The new staff member's clinical competencies would be reviewed and the final decision would rest with the staff. If staff nurses were self-governed and responsible for hiring and firing, would they have the right to strike?

AUTHORITY

Authority derives in large part from organizational power. It is the right to take actions. Formal or official authority is vested in the position held (e.g. Director of Nursing). Formal authority clearly delineates subordinate and superordinate positions. Authority of legitimacy connotes authority by title only. In this case, subordinates defer to authority. In other words, the staff nurse may write an anecdote about another staff nurse's performance and defer to the legitimate authority empowered by position to make the decision. Staff nurses may alternately try to exercise authority as a group independent of legitimate authority. This is where confrontation and collective bargaining emerge. Confrontation and collective bargaining require that the nurse leader develop collaborative communication skills in order to develop collegial relationships.

INFLUENCE

To influence others we must view each individual as unique. Certain basic attitudes toward each individual should be adopted:

1. Each person brings a lifelong history of coping mechanisms and problem-solving skills to a given situation. Experiences are drawn from adverse and hostile situations brought about by virtue of ethnicity, cultural background, race, religious affiliation, socioeconomic status, geographical background—rural versus urban, inner urban versus suburban. We must accept and respect the history that each person brings to a relationship.

2. Each person's history reveals a special identity, lifestyle, and skill. Do you take the time to try to get to know the nurses you are working with? How many children do they have? What are their outside interests? What makes them tick as a person? Suddenly professional differences arise and you're faced with a confrontation. If personal compatibilities are previously established, confrontations can be more easily resolved with the personal relationship remaining intact. That unique personal background creates a special identity that goes beyond professional conflict.

3. The observable human response is innate and adaptive and responses are appropriate reactions given certain social situations. If a nurse leader sets out to resolve a conflict with a physician bearing an openly aggressive posture, the physician is not going to hear what the nurse is saying. However, if the situation is clearly understood by both parties and each knows the other's emotional response to the situation, the relationship has a better chance of succeeding and the conflict has a better chance of being resolved.

4. Differences in expected and observed actions have a logical meaning. A nurse is expected to follow physicians' orders but is observed to question, challenge, and interpret the orders based on nursing assessment. When this behavior is demonstrated consistently at a high level competency, the differences have a logical meaning.

5. Differences need not cause problems; they can be challenging. They can even be an asset. The nurse who demonstrates clinical excellence in her challenging and questioning of others will demonstrate substantial differences in quality patient care outcomes and will be viewed as an asset.

6. You must want to hear what the other person has to say. Active listening is concentrating on and responding to the facts and feelings the other person is conveying. Respond to feelings in a manner that is comfortable for you and expect that certain emotions will be present. Try to deal with emotions in a way that will not interfere with communication.

7. You must attempt to genuinely accept the other person's feelings however different they may be from your own. Emotions are not negotiable or subject to dispute. If a person is angry, hostile, or belligerent, you learn to accept the behavior as a symptom of a problem and not a personal attack.

8. Trust both an individual's capability to handle problems and emotions and his desire to seek equitable solutions. No one really enjoys disruptive feelings and problems which interfere with positive working relationships.

9. Remember, emotions and thoughts are subject to change: indifference

can change to responsibility; annoyance to acceptance; discouragement to hope; frustration to resolution.

10. Mutual benefit and appropriate management of our own feelings usually occurs when sensitive listening and open, honest responding takes place. We should strive to disagree about principles without reacting to the person and creating a permanent barrier. We have a right to disagree intellectually. That doesn't mean that we cannot continue to work in a collegial way with the individual, whether extra or interdepartmentally, within the nurse/nurse, nurse/physician, or nurse/administrator relationship.

These basic attitudes for collaborative communications and a brief overview of power and authority should assist nurses in the development of strategies for overcoming barriers to intercollegial relationships.

REFERENCE

1. Fiedler, F., Chemers, M., Mahar, L. *Improving Leadership Effectiveness: The Leader Match Concept.* New York: Wiley, 1976.

The Inconsistent Supply of Professionally Qualified Nurses

by Margaret L. McClure
Director of Nursing
Maimonides Medical Center
Brooklyn, New York

One of the major problems confronting any group that sets out to discuss the notion of an ALL-RN staff is the immediate realization that there is not a single operational definition of the term registered nurse. It becomes clear from the outset that today's registered nurse cannot be described as an individual with a set of particular characteristics but can rather be one of several types of persons. I am alluding, of course, to the variety of tracks of educational preparation that the nurse might have pursued en route to licensure. At present, these consist of the diploma, the associate degree, the baccalaureate degree, the general master's degree, and the recently established professional doctorate in nursing[1].

One of nursing's tasks is to address the problem of the inconsistent supply of professionally qualified nurses. Given the state of our basic educational affairs, it becomes necessary to define just what the words "professionally qualified nurses" will mean for the purpose of discussion. For many nursing leaders in the country, the accepted, albeit heatedly debated, definition of the professional in nursing is one prepared with a minimum of a baccalaureate degree in nursing. While such a definition is supported throughout the nursing literature, its acceptance, particularly by those with less than baccalaureate education, has been tentative at best. It would probably be safe to say that all registered nurses in this country consider themselves professionals, regardless of their educational preparation.

REGISTERED NURSE AS PROFESSIONAL

The notion that all registered nurses are professionals receives a good deal of support in the "real world." It is certainly given credence by the fact that all types of graduates without exception take the same state board examination and on passing the exam, receive the same license; in many states the license itself bears the words "registered professional nurse." It is important to keep in mind that the license relates directly to a nursing practice act in each state. These acts spell out a legal definition of professional nursing that describes the scope of practice of the practitioner to whom the license is issued. Since all RNs, regardless of preparation, are covered by the same definition, it becomes quite clear that every registered nurse has the legal right to the title of professional.

Further, employers contribute to this point of view by offering identical positions with identical titles and, for all practical purposes, identical salaries to the various graduates. Thus, our lack of discrimination in the areas of licensure, job description, and salary lends support to the idea that all RNs are professionals. As a result, a certain amount of leveling tends to occur in our collective minds.

Indications, however, suggest that employers are finding significant differences between graduates of the various programs[2] and are beginning to reflect these in their hiring and promotional policies[3]. These changes are undoubtedly due to the increasing complexity in recent years of all aspects of health-care delivery with the resultant requirement that nurses have more sophisticated preparation than their predecessors. The demands by the various accrediting and certifying agencies alone bear witness to the fact that nursing can no longer survive with individuals who have only technical competence; intellectual skills are being taxed to the utmost in service agencies and this emphasis will undoubtedly increase in the years to come. This development has led the American Nurses Association to once again address the serious educational issues currently facing the profession.

While the stance of the professional association has appeared ambiguous at times, two clear actions, taken by two distinctly different houses of delegates, are of importance with regard to the definition of the professional nurse. In 1966 approval was given to the statement entitled *Educational Preparation for Nurse Practitioners & Assistants to Nurses* that had been published by the Commission on Education in 1965. In essence, this report called for two basic educational preparations for the practice of nursing; professional, prepared at the baccalaureate level and technical, prepared at the associate degree level[4]. Unfortunately, no timetable for implementation was included in the position paper and over the years it continued to be alluded to as the profession's goal for the future. At the 1978 ANA convention in Hawaii, however, the organization passed a resolution calling for baccalaureate preparation in nursing to become the minimum level of preparation for new professional nurses by 1985. Included in the pronouncement was strong support for a grandfather clause that would permit all nurses licensed or eligible for licensure prior to 1985 to continue practicing as registered nurses, regardless of educational preparation. This action represents a giant step forward; however, without changes in the laws related to such a proposal, it remains questionable as to whether such a stance taken by the professional association can be placed into operation.

PATIENT CARE/STAFFING MODELS

Today we face the task of taking the foregoing material into account as we confront the problems of (1) the inconsistent supply of all RNs, and (2) the inconsistent supply of baccalaureate degree nurses.

In any case, regardless of which of the two questions one may choose to address, there is one practical issue that confronts all of the professions, including nursing; that is the geographical maldistribution of qualified practitioners. In some areas, baccalaureate graduates are almost nonexistent and diploma and associate degree graduates are in frighteningly short supply. In others the supply is erratic and unpredictable. In a few more fortunate locations the supply is available and predictable[5]. The challenge, then, is to design patient care/staffing models that take into account the constraints that the supply problem imposes. A few models, well-known in acute care settings, come to mind.

One familiar model is team nursing. This particular approach was designed to maximize the impact of the professional nurse's unique skills and knowledge. Theoretically, the professional was to function as team leader and in this way influence the care that all members of the team delivered. Clearly this model could be very helpful in situations where professionals are in short supply and where much of the direct care is rendered by nonprofessional staff. However, many of us have become disenchanted with team nursing because the results have not been as favorable as had been originally hoped. The reasons for this have been many, but the crux of the problem seems to center on such factors as unreasonable work loads for team leaders and too little real supervision of team members.

As somewhat of an aside, we must acknowledge the extreme difficulty that direct supervision to nonprofessionnals in nursing poses because of the intimate nature of the work. Much of the care that is rendered must, of necessity, be done behind closed curtains or doors, with the result that supervision automatically becomes more general than one might hope.

A second model that has received considerable attention and acclaim is that of primary nursing. Such a model might lend itself well to the future plan for the educational preparation of two levels of practitioners. In this case the primary nurse role could be filled by the professional and the associate nurse role by the graduate of the associate degree program. This would require a supply situation in which adequate numbers of both types of nurses would be available. The negative features of such a model are related to aspects of the individual nurse's career. First, it assumes that all professional nurses, including novices, are competent to function as primary nurses; clearly this is not the case in many situations. Second, it does not allow for clinical career advancement. Each type of nurse would enter the work setting in a particular role and stay there.

A third model, then, seems to be in order, one that utilizes primary nursing in a more realistic manner with room for career growth. This would call for the seasoned, clinically competent nurse to act as the primary nurse while the less experienced nurse functioned in the associate nurse role. Clearly into such an arrangement are built rewards for clinical expertise, offering the individual nurse an opportunity for advancement. The supply problems with this particular model, are, of course, enormous and represent a very real constraint on placing such an approach into operation in most settings.

A discussion such as this is most productive if it begins by looking very carefully at the problems related to the supply of qualified professional nurses. Then, specific actions needed to attack these problems can be explored. In such a venture it is very important to think big and not be content to address only "what is" but also to give thoughtful attention to what might be. Perhaps through such a discussion we might be able to clarify what we see as our needs in service settings and develop the planning strategies required to meet those needs.

REFERENCES

1.   Case Western Reserve to introduce ND degree, *Nursing Outlook,* 26(7):412–413, 1978.
2.   Howell, F.J. Employers evaluations of new graduates, *Nursing Outlook,* 1978, 26(7):446–451, 1978.
3.   Hillsmith, K.E. From RN to BSN: Student perceptions, *Nursing Outlook,* 1978, 26(2):98–102, 1978.
4.   American Nurses Association. *Educational Preparation for Nurse Practitioners & Assistants to Nurses,* ANA, 1965.
5.   Sloan, F.A. *The geographic distribution of nurses and public policy.* Bethesda, Maryland. U.S. Department of Health, Education & Welfare, 1975.

Existing Nursing Management Structures

by June Werner

One major obstacle in the implementation of the ALL-RN staff is existing management structures. Historically, like every other enterprise, nursing developed a structure that was assumed would get the job done. Prior to World War II, the case method serviced that purpose. The patient knew his nurse, she was there at least twelve hours a day, sometimes six or seven days a week and often went home with him.

With the advent of the technology that followed the war, the industrial model was introduced to hospitals and in particular to nursing at a time when the availability of RNs was very low. The management response to this dilemma evolved with little input from nurses. Hospital administrators, assisted by industrial engineers, took it upon themselves to find solutions. The question could not have been asked, "What does the patient need?" The question from the hospital administrators and their industrial consultants was, "How do we get the work done?" Nursing, to the hospital administrators and industrial engineers, was "a bundle of tasks" to be done for patients. They had no idea that it involved a process, the outcome of whose quality depended on sequence, continuity, and the clinical competence of the nurse. Furthermore, nursing at that time played a minimal role in clinical or hospital decision making and certainly had no behavioral model for autonomy or even assertiveness.

Given these conditions at a time when medical technology entered an explosive era, it is perhaps not surprising that the succeeding events took place. What *is* distressing is that it has taken us so long to reconstruct models that are acceptable to the world of patients, hospitals, and health care. Some of this is understandable if we take into account that as we became aware of the need for professional autonomy, then learned to articulate the premises of nursing, the era of great fiscal constraints was almost upon us.

ACCOUNTABILITY FOR OUTCOMES OF CARE

One way of looking at administrative structure is to look at the nature of nursing as a clinical practice, as we view it today, and at the accountability inherent in the profession and subsequently how the existing structure effects the transfer of accountability.

Accountability for the outcomes of care of any patient is designed to facilitate optimal recovery and an acceptable hospital experience which is safe, consistent, and planned to take into account the patient's individuality. Our assumption is that this can best be accomplished by a process that includes *assessment, planning* on the basis of that assessment, the *implementation* of those plans, and monitoring the effectiveness of those plans and the patient status by continuous *evaluation.* The governing board of the hospital has the accountability for the care of patients in the facility. They delegate their accountability to physicians and nurses for care in their respective domains. In very few places the accountability for nursing care is delegated through physicians to nurses. That is not a contemporary view or pattern. The *administration* of nursing and medicine is delegated through a chief executive officer. The nursing administrator then delegates her accountability, which is sustained accountability, to her assistants for each clinical area. They are called supervisors, coordinators, or directors. In larger settings there is another layer of assistants—assistant directors—to whom the supervisors report. The supervisors then delegate their accountability to head nurses who have the accountability for nursing care of the population of patients on their unit and to each individual patient.

It may help to look at a specific patient. Our patient is a middle-aged, hard-working female professional with an administrative position. She has been admitted to the hospital for (1) a cholecystectomy and (2) to rule out mild situational hypertension.

In most existing management structures, the head nurse delegates the care of each patient on the unit to members of the staff. This is done in myriad ways.

1. Using the *functional method,* the patient may be cared for by a number of people, each person doing something different for the patient. The staff person who bathes the patient and makes his bed may be a different employee each day. This person may also do the patient's treatments, but not always. In some systems that same person may do some teaching. Any of these care givers may be on-the-job trained staff.

2. The *team method* has been the prevailing way of providing care in this country for more than twenty years. The team members may be nurses and/or nursing assistants. In most teams there is a team leader who is a nurse. Presumably the accountability for the nursing care of the patients on the team has been given to the leader who then passes it on to assistants, to LPNs and

Figure 1. What the Patient* Gets in Most Existing Management Structures

(How is the case "managed" in terms of this patient's* nursing care?)

RN₂ 🔲 LPN₃ ▥ NA₅ ▦	NIGHTS	EVENINGS	DAYS
Sun.	NA₆	LPN₃	
Mon.	NA₇	RN₂	RN₁
Tues.	NA₇	LPN₄	RN₁
Wed.	NA₇	LPN₄	NA₉
Thurs.	NA₈	LPN₅	NA₉
Fri.	NA₆	LPN₅	NA₉
Sat.			NA₁₀

*Patient is middle aged, hard-working female professional with administrative position. Having Cholecystectomy. Rule out mild situational hypertension.

nursing aides. It is the LPN and aides who provide most of the direct care, each for a period of eight hours. The next day the assignment may very well change. For whatever reason the care-giver is a new and different person, most usually a nonprofessional, as the patient recovers. All the nonprofessional can do for our patient is limited by a one-year technical education base and experience, whatever that may be, plus in some cases on-the-job training.

Figure 1 illustrates the impact of the existing management structure on the patient. You will remember that our patient is going to have a cholecystectomy. She is admitted on a busy Sunday afternoon and is cared for by an RN who has the responsibility for admissions. That night she has some difficulty sleeping despite medication and finds she has forgotten to ask some pertinent questions about her post-operative course. The nursing assistant on nights cannot answer her questions and suggests she wait until morning when an RN is available. There is little opportunity to ask questions in the morning since she has her pre-operative medication almost as soon as she awakens.

During a five and one half day hospital stay she has ten care givers, only two of whom are RNs. Our patient will have spent 144 hours in the hospital. She will have had about twenty-six hours of direct nursing care, only four hours given by an RN.

Who is accountable for the nursing care of our patient? Our middle-aged woman executive is having major surgery and is perhaps more than a little worried about her situational hypertension. Maybe the answer is, the nursing staff who's taking care of her. Everyone?

If we view accountability in the professional sense, it is most graphic if we use the architectural model. No one pays architects for simply going to their office every day and doing whatever architects do. Architects are paid for, and their reputations depend on, the outcomes of their practice. This accountability is not shared with all the assistants who help the architects accomplish their goals. It is the *architect's* building and it is the *architect* who must live with the outcomes.

Is it reasonable to think that nursing, a professional discipline, should be any different? Are we accountable for the outcomes of our practice? Does nursing owe this same kind of accountability to its consumers? Can a group of well-meaning hospital employees with different amounts of training, with diverse expectations, *collectively* be accountable? If they cannot, can the head nurse be accountable? It really doesn't seem humanly possible. For years, nursing administrators have felt that this was acceptable. They slept better at night because they felt they provided nurses with supervisors, "just to make sure," to "check." If that system was ever workable, it is no longer.

GENERIC MODEL OF CLINICAL MANAGEMENT

We are in an era where we must consider sophisticated diagnostic and

Figure 2. A Clinical Management Structure

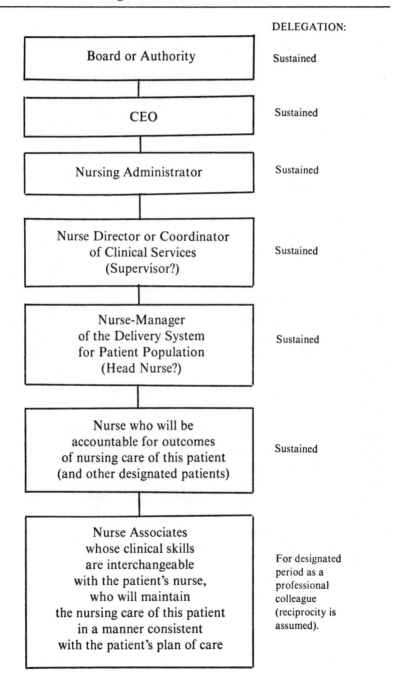

treatment modalities, high acuity, shortened length of patient stays. This, compounded by quality assurance and concerns about liability, means that accountability must be placed on the competent care givers who are educated and licensed in terms of the expectations of accountability.

There are probably many alternatives. Figure 2 is a view of the generic model of a clinical management service. Authority is vested in the board. Although the *administrative* component is transferred to the chief executive officer, the *clinical* accountability bypasses him and is passed from the board to the nursing administrator for the clinical practice of nursing in the institution. The nursing administrator delegates her accountability to the directors or coordinators, sometimes supervisors, of the different clinical services, who pass it on to the nurse-manager of the delivery system for a designated population of patients. This may be the head nurse or an alternate, more contemporary title.

Accountability is now delegated to the patient's nurse who has the accountability for the outcomes of nursing care for that patient. The nurse is assisted by her associate nurses, similarly if not identically trained, holding the same license to practice. If and when hospitals progress to the point where support services are sufficiently responsive that adaptations for care are not required because of absent or wrong equipment and supplies, where all physicians can agree on diagnostic and treatment modalities and where nurses are tenured, experienced, and turnover problems no longer exist, then I believe we could eliminate one if not two of these layers. While most of us feel that at least one of the levels are necessary, each person in their separate setting must decide what guarantees are necessary.

The patient has a nurse with associates to share the care; the associate's clinical skills are assumed to be interchangeable with the patient's nurse. Together the nurse and associate maintain the nursing care of this patient in a manner consistent with the patient's plan of care. We know lots of middle-aged women executives who might have a cholecystectomy and could conceivably have situational hypertension. Wouldn't it seem advisable for that patient to have ALL-RNs caring for her?

In Figure 3 the invisible management is as obscure as it was in the existing structure. The six care givers, all RNs, are sufficiently self-assured to make the patient feel no need for visible management.

In Figure 4 the time span of the six RNs who care for our patient is depicted. The consistency is clear. Nursing practice in terms of this patient is very different from that depicted in the last example. All six care givers can practice in terms of nursing process.

They know how to acquire a data base, they understand the need to plan, and the importance of the patient's input. They can implement plans, not merely follow orders and protocols. They adapt, then, with the patient, to best meet this particular patient's needs. They can elevate the status of the patient

Figure 3. An Alternative: What the Patient* Gets in Most Existing Management Structures

(How is the case "managed" in terms of this patient's nursing care?)

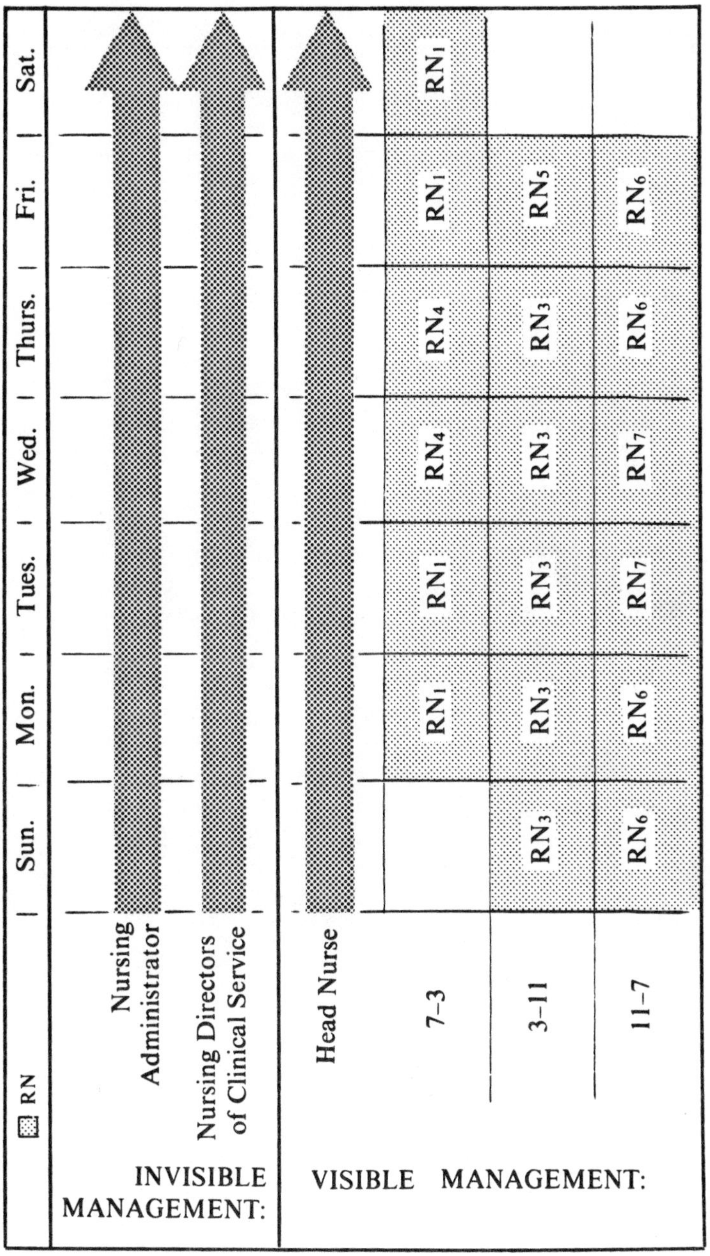

| RN | Sun. | Mon. | Tues. | Wed. | Thurs. | Fri. | Sat. |

INVISIBLE MANAGEMENT:
- Nursing Administrator
- Nursing Directors of Clinical Service

VISIBLE MANAGEMENT:
- Head Nurse

	Sun.	Mon.	Tues.	Wed.	Thurs.	Fri.	Sat.
7–3	RN₃	RN₁	RN₁	RN₄	RN₄	RN₁	RN₁
3–11	RN₆	RN₃	RN₃	RN₃	RN₃	RN₅	
11–7		RN₆	RN₇	RN₇	RN₆	RN₆	

*Patient is middle aged, hard-working female professional with administrative position. Having Cholecystectomy. Rule out mild situational hypertension.

Figure 4. An Alternative: What the Patient* Gets in Most Existing Management Structures

---

(How is the case "managed" in terms of this patient's* nursing care?)

RN_6 ▨	NIGHTS	EVENINGS	DAYS
Sun.	RN_5	RN_2	
Mon.	RN_6	RN_2	RN_1
Tues.	RN_6	RN_2	RN_1
Wed.	RN_5	RN_2	RN_3
Thurs.	RN_5	RN_2	RN_3
Fri.	RN_5	RN_4	RN_1
Sat.			RN_1

*Patient is middle aged, hard-working female professional with administrative position. Having Cholecystectomy. Rule out mild situational hypertension.

and the quality of care, validate with each other and in the best of all worlds, learn from each other. This alternative structure can only work when nursing is perceived as a clinical discipline and all the non-nursing duties are accomplished by other personnel. It is simply too expensive to have nurses doing the tasks that can be more economically done by nonprofessionals. This is a problem for management to solve. Nurses must keep an open mind and a reality orientation toward clinical practice in order to help with the solutions.

We have been looking at existing management structures and at an alternative to improved care using an ALL-RN staff. If we are to change such structures, most of us cannot accomplish this spontaneously or by declaring it a reasonable alternative and causing it to happen over night. In new facilities few of us would consider anything but an ALL-RN staff. In existing institutions, however, it is not easy to bring about unless there is a carefully planned mechanism developed for the change. The obvious rationale for making this change is the ongoing needs of the patient. When it can be demonstrated that the needs of a given patient population are such that they can best be met by professional nurses, it is time to implement the plan, on the basis of safety and cost effectiveness.

CHANGING THE SYSTEM

The next two figures illustrate the experience of Hospital X, a 500-bed teaching hospital in the Midwest. From 1972 through 1977, number of RNs in the hospital increased from 33 percent to 73 percent and they continue to plan for a further increase. You will note that in the HAS reports, the comparisons show fewer hours paid per patient day, and in two groups of patients and less salary expense per patient day in medical-surgical units. I share some notes with you from the nursing administrator at Hospital X. "Changing the structure meant changing the system. We shared the rationale for this with our staff. One of the outcomes of this was that a good number of our LPNs and our nursing assistants went back to school to acquire a graduate nurse education. The personnel department opened up other positions in the hospital as we looked for positions for the staff being displaced. No one was simply terminated to make room for the RNs. All budget change requests to exchange nonprofessionals for professionals were well documented in terms of program, patient needs, fiscal accountability, and a need to find suitable employment for the nonprofessional staff member being replaced." We must face the fact that many of our existing structures are obsolete, meeting neither the needs of our patients nor responding pragmatically to the clinical competence of today's professional nurse. In the past when it became necessary to change our management structures, nursing allowed other disciplines to do it for us. This time we need to develop a plan ourselves with appropriate input as needed. We know the needs of patients and we know the capacity of today's nurse. Our job is to create a workable model for blending both.

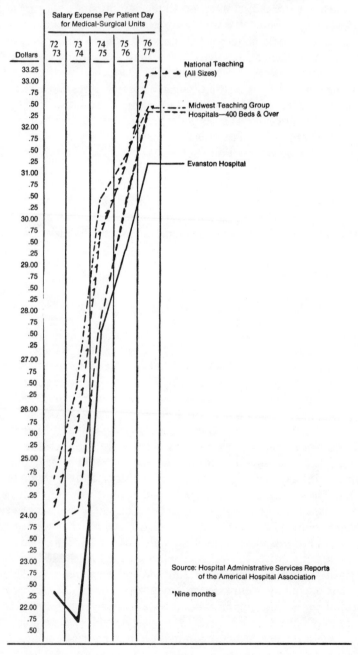

	Nursing Hours Paid Per Patient Day for All Nursing Units					Nursing Hours Paid Per Patient Day for Medical-Surgical Units				
	72 73	73 74	74 75	75 76	76 77*	72 73	73 74	74 75	75 76	76 77*

Source: Hospital Administrative Service Reports of the American Hospital Association

*Nine months

— · — · — Midwest Teaching Group

— — — Hospitals—400 Beds & Over

— — → National Teaching (All Sizes)

———— Evanston Hospital

Power Limitations for Nurses Initiating Change

by Luther Christman

Presented here are some personal observations regarding barriers to initiating change in the field of nursing. Once such barriers are identified, strategies can be devised to overcome them. Generally speaking, the principal problems facing nursing lie at the macro level. There is no critical professional problem in each health-care facility; the problem lies with the external reference group and the state-of-the-art of the field as it is perceived by those with whom we must work. The perspective I take in the remarks that follow is that we are the outcome of how the issues are perceived nationally.

DEFINING NURSING

One of the major issues that divides us as a profession is the definition of the technical and professional nurse. Technical and professional nursing as an entity cannot be quantitatively defined. Cognitive and psychomotor skills can be quantified, but restricting our definition to the skills we arrive at a conception of nursing limited only by the knowledge system of the nurses. This leads to the troublesome, unresolved conflict over who and what is a nurse—two, three, or four years of preparation for practice. Until we can define ourselves to the rest of the world, we remain in a tenuous position. Physical therapists, occupational therapists, dentists and physicians are easily identifiable to the world at large. Nurses are not so easily categorized. There is great variation as others see us, and as long as we have such resistance to a resolution to this conflict, nursing as a profession will remain at a standstill.

Another major issue, one that holds us back more than almost any other, is the complete separation of education and service. We are the only group of professionals that seems intent on making it impossible for either education or service to get its work done.

USING THE EXPERIENCED NURSE IN CLINICAL PRACTICE

Another major issue that immobilizes our profession is that we are the only clinical profession that doesn't regularly use its most gifted persons in the care of patients. All of the direct nursing care is done almost entirely by young graduates. These inexperienced nurses form the public's image of the profession, and not those persons several layers removed from direct nursing care. Most of us would undoubtedly prefer to be cared for by a physician who has been practicing for twenty years rather than someone in her or his first year of clinical practice. Certainly if we want advice and help from a clinical psychologist or if we want good dental care, we go to an experienced clinician. Patients don't have that same experience with nurses. In nursing, we assume that after two or three years of experience, we should move away from direct care. We've never established a career structure of clinical competence in nursing as it exists in other health-care professions. Only recently have we begun to see some nurses with graduate preparation and experience involved deeply in patient care, but that is still a fairly sporadic occurrence. As long as the youth must carry the profession, we will not move forward.

Some length of time is required to saturate the knowledge systems and become efficient in the implementation of those systems. That time requirement has been absent in nursing in the post-World War II era. Prior to World War II, experienced nurses entered private practice and the inexperienced and less competent nurses practiced in hospitals. We relinquished the system of direct payment to nurses when we moved from private practice to bureaucracy.

Following World War II, Senator Hill, a Democrat from Alabama, and Senator Burton, a Republican from Ohio, sponsored a hospital construction bill, later referred to as the Hill/Burton Bill. Being a bipartisan bill, it sailed through Congress. Lawmakers often simplistically and falsely assume that if you pass a law, all the problems disappear. The hospital construction act was passed to provide easier access to hospitals for all citizens. Unfortunately, all the hospitals constructed as a result of this legislation were built in the wrong places at the wrong times for the wrong reasons. The more rural the community the more likely it would get a hospital.

The nation, on the other hand, was moving from a rural to an urban society. Congressmen presumed that nurses and physicians would gravitate to the hospitals, regardless of location. Twenty years later, realizing their mistake, Congress enacted the manpower bill to train nurses, physicians and other hospital personnel. By that time the health-care system was in hopeless disarray.

One scarce resource was trained hospital administrators. There were only a few programs in hospital administration in the country before World War II. Hospitals were built as rapidly as possible yet few were managed by competent administrators. Boards of directors, searching for other means of managing the hospitals, looked to industry and began recruiting corporate executives. These executives brought their systems engineers and other management tools, concluding that a patient is a patient just as a bicycle is a bicycle. If you wish to manufacture bicycles, you assign specific tasks to specialists and the bicycles are easily assembled. The same notion seemed appropriate for care of patients.

At that time, few nurses in the country desired or gave much thought to advanced preparation. They were pulled by the tide of war and following it, the great pressure to staff. Private practice nursing was disrupted by the war as many nurses joined the Army and Navy Nurse Corps. With the hospital system expanding in all directions after the war, few nurses were sufficiently educated to assume leadership positions and assert "we won't be all things to all people, we'll just do nursing." Instead, they tried to run the hospitals that were expanding faster than they could be managed. Being undertrained, nurses were easily enthralled by the systems engineers who concluded, "it takes this much activity to do a bed bath, just get an aide in here—a bath is a bath." Nurses, unable to cope with all this information and being so undertrained in comparison with physicians, hospital administrators, systems engineers and others moving into the system, were swept along with the tide.

One large eastern university that assumed a principal role in advanced education for nurses decided to forego the training of clinicians. Instead, graduate education was offered in administration or education, neither of which had anything to do with the practice of nursing. These graduates were neither fish nor fowl. They were not fully trained administrators nor fully trained nurses at a professional level comparable to their colleagues in other health-care professions. These simultaneous occurrences led us to where we are now.

When the systems engineers introduced task specialization studies leading to team nursing, the entire pattern of nurses removed from direct care of patients commenced. The engineers insisted that to be cost effective the least expensive health-care workers should be next to the patient. The data that my colleagues and I have accumulated suggest that the engineers asked the wrong questions and gathered inappropriate data. Aides are more costly than a staff comprised entirely of registered nurses. Our data of several years past suggest that nurses with master's degrees would be the most cost effective per unit of care. Nursing has never followed that pattern, partly because we separated education from service contrary to other clinical professions.

UNITING AND EXTENDING THE PROFESSION

The enormous competition at the national level between the nursing organizations is another problem facing our profession. Each seems to want to outdo the other and, if they can, cause the other to stumble a bit. It is very interesting to note that nurses who are members of both or more than two organizations all act differently and vote differently in those organizations when they are in respective sessions and often vote at odds with each other and themselves. I've never been quite able to understand that behavior, but it appears to happen regularly.

Our complete lack of lobbying strength vis a vis other professional organization is another impediment to accumulating power. This does not mean that we have no lobbying strength but in comparison with the strength of the AHA and the AMA we do poorly.

Lack of a scholarly record is another weakness in our profession. Nurse researchers frequently quote the research of other scientists and professionals, but nursing research is rarely quoted in the literature of other professions. We don't have the record of scholarship needed to influence other groups to the degree that our statements are accepted with a high degree of credibility. These issues are not new but they certainly are vital to the growth of power.

THE QUESTION OF PROFESSIONAL ACCOUNTABILITY

Lack of accountability in the nursing care system warrants examination. To give an example, we studied continuity of care at four nonteaching general hospitals a number of years ago. It was nonexistent, even on a daily basis. It was as though the patients were cared for by three distinctly different hospital systems each day. Each nursing shift operated differently and the patients had to adjust to the nursing staff, not the nurses to the patients. In our conversations with patients, they remarked similarly that when the day nurses are on duty, the work is done one way; the evening nurses do it another way; and at night, something new comes up. Every day a different nurse was assigned to a given patient. No nurse wanted the same patient for two consecutive days because the same assignment was too boring: "I had cranky Mrs. Jones yesterday, today you have cranky Mrs. Jones." No one thought about why Mrs. Jones was cranky. She was cranky because she did not know what was happening to her. She wanted some stability in the system and it was not there. The nurses never looked at the situation from the perspective of the patient. They blamed the patient instead of examining their own actions.

The various regulatory agencies, governmental or voluntary, present a great burden to implementing change. We just completed a certificate of need review for modernization of our hospital. A seventy-five million dollar wing is planned to replace outmoded facilities. We finally received approval after several months of intense negotiation. However, the first design of the hospital was rejected out of hand by a state planning official.

The objections raised were based on a number of factors, including questions about the appropriateness of nurses involved in the design process. We were pleased with the architectural plans because they were heavily influenced by the nursing staff. One of the principal reasons for resistance appears to have been based on a misconception and a misinterpretation of "primary nursing." In the point of view of the state official, primary nursing was "coddling patients" and with some vehemence it was made clear that "the state is not in the business of coddling patients."

Rather than give the subject the thought it deserved, the reviewer fell back on certain stereotypes. He wanted it redesigned because the best way to give care to his mind was to find out which nurse on the staff was the best back rubber and she would rub everyone's back. Find out which nurse could give pills best and have her give pills to everyone in the hospital. It took time to reach agreement about our original design. When I'm commenting about government and other regulatory agencies that keep us from getting our work done, it is not idle chatter. Nurses must work toward neutralizing these forces, both by clarifying their practice and by active participation in the politicizing process.

REAPING THE BENEFITS OF CHANGE

When I first arrived at Rush, between 80 and 90 percent of the letters received in our hospital from patients complained of the poor nursing care and the impersonal attitude of the nursing staff. If we get one of those letters now once in three months, it's rare. Over 99 percent of the letters received about nursing are highly complimentary. The change correlated with the move to primary nursing and the preponderance of registered nurses on the staff.

The physicians have had the greatest turnaround. When I first arrived at Rush there was a physician who had the reputation of never complimenting anyone. He was an enormously competent physician himself, a very good clinician; he had a large practice and was very effective at managing patients but he expected the same from everyone and most people didn't meet his standards of performance. About once a week during my first year he used to drop by my office to make negative observations and comments. During my second year he backed off a little and did not complain as regularly. One day recently he rapped at my door and asked if he could interrupt me for a moment. He said, "I just want to tell you that six years ago this place was a bunch of men in white coats running around writing orders and today it's a hospital." Physician turnaround is enormous when nurses perform in good clinical fashion.

When we were looking at continuity of care in a major university hospital, we also looked at tender loving care as it's defined in the literature. In two years of daily data gathering, none was detected. Team nursing was in operation in the system at that time. When we asked each nurse (and we did regularly) how much tender care was being given to the patient, we were told by each nurse such care was given all day long. We asked patients the same question. Their response was zero. Who was right? The patients. This empathy, interest in the patient, dealing with the patient's anxiety, the giving of social and emotional support is often more myth than reality.

To give an example of what we declared was not tender loving care, consider the usual parade in a university hospital. The long coats, the short coats, and women in white making rounds. As physicians and nurses always do, they sit on both sides of the bed talking as if the patient isn't there, using language that no one but them understands. In one instance, there was a patient whom I knew was doing quite well because I was on the unit every day. He was getting ready to go home when the team passed by; he called me over and said he was all upset because he thought that all that language was a code so that he wouldn't understand that he was having a relapse and was actually getting worse. He didn't feed badly until they talked around, not to, him. Then, because of all the strange language, he was sure they were keeping something from him.

He had an average education. He was a blue-collar worker and probably thought in concrete terms. Part of the ground rules for the research I conducted was that I wouldn't intervene with the patients. I could only suggest to him that he ask one of the nurses what their discussion meant. Eventually, the young nurse came by with a big tray of medication and the patient asked her if she wouldn't be kind enough to stop so he could ask her some questions as he was disturbed by her previous conversation and wanted some answers. Before he could ask the first question, she stood there and said, "You see all of these medications. I've got to get them all out to all the patients on time, you don't want me to stop now, do you?" He just folded up his tent and said, no. Then she said something that was very kind, "As soon as I am not busy, I'll come back and sit with you." When do you think she came back? She was never "not busy" and he just hung there all day. When I talked with her afterward, she was quite upset with me. She said, you saw how kind I was to him and how busy I was. What else would he or you want in that situation? She still couldn't see the consequences of her behavior.

We found that these incidents of social politeness were considered to be tender loving care. Many such variations on this theme occurred daily over the two years of the study. This may have been an unusual hospital but the same thing was evident when we studied four nonteaching community hospitals later. The four-hospital study came after the university-hospital study and there was no difference in the way nurses saw patients in either university hospitals or community hospitals. Without patient support, nurses lose power. When we build patient constituency, we build power. That's how a lot of physicians get power. Patients think that physicians heal them; they like them. I'm sure that in many hospitals today, nurses have more power and influence in the work situation. A high degree of patient satisfaction with service rendered by a group gives an enormous bargaining power.

The Cost of ALL-RN Staffing

by Marguerite L. Burt

Because RN salaries are usually higher than those of LVNs and other categories of nursing staff, it's easy to assume that an ALL-RN staff would cost more. Of course, there is much more to staffing cost than salary, but salary is a good indicator of total cost and our experience at the VA Hospital in San Antonio, Texas, shows that an ALL-RN staff does not cost more! We have not yet studied such other cost factors as on-the-job training, recruitment budgets, turnover rates, supervisory demands, counseling time, continuing education, or behavioral problems. But, we are convinced that data about these other factors would further support use of an ALL-RN nursing staff.

The Audie L. Murphy Veterans Administration Hospital opened October 29, 1973, and I joined the staff in March of that year to plan and implement its nursing service. The hospital now has a capacity for 700 patients with bed sections for medical, surgical, psychiatric, and rehabilitation services. There are special care units for coronary care, medical intensive care, surgical intensive care, and for special diagnostic treatments. The ambulatory care area (outpatient) is funded for 167,000 visits in 1978 and there are three satellite clinics. There are approved residency training programs in medicine, surgery, dentistry, anesthesiology, neurology, pathology, psychiatry, radiology, and audiology. The VA Hospital is a major part of the University of Texas Health Science Center and is located in the same medical complex. Nursing students affiliate with us from the University of Texas School of Nursing, Incarnate Word College, and San Antonio Community College. In addition, RNs are also assigned to such other programs as the day hospital, the day treatment center, radiology, and the cardiac catheter lab. They are also assigned as nurse practitioners to health maintenance clinics, in leukophoresis, infection control, and community nursing. In establishing the nursing service, I found many supportive elements. The director and assistant director expected the chief nurse and her staff to establish and implement an outstanding service, and each of them was receptive to new ideas. I was able to recruit outstanding associates and our "dreams for a truly different organization" began to get set down on paper. In addition to hospital management's strong support and guidance, we had encouragement from the Director of Nursing Service in the Central Office in Washington, a Freisen-type building that had nurse servers built in, and plans to install the unit dose system and a medication additive program run by pharmacy personnel. Plans also included a complete twenty-four hour Supply, Processing and Delivery System (SPD), and other supporting services (such as medical administration and building management) that would assume their functions on the nursing units, permitting nursing personnel to nurse patients, not things.

A major supportive factor was the freedom to set up our organization from scratch. This was an exciting experience that led us to an organization design based on the primary nurse model of care using an ALL-RN staff. The activation plan for the hospital had been developed in 1972 by the assistant director. The plan included a nursing staff of 617 people (see Table 1).

In developing our staffing plan, we set several guidelines: the RN would be the direct care provider (primary and associate nurses); if we ever decided to include another category, we would consider the LVN so that only registered or licensed staff would provide care; and we would remain with an ALL-RN staff until we knew on which units *carefully selected* LVNs could be utilized safely. Our basic strategy was to trade two LVN or nursing assistant positions for one RN position. This went on unit-by-unit as we activated, and was possible on all units except psychiatry. The activation plan allowed only five RNs for a thirty bed unit, too few to provide a nursing care coordinator and RN supervisor on each tour. So we had to ask for an exception, bringing RN staff on the psychiatric units to fifteen. We hoped to recover these extra positions, and succeeded, as we staffed other units. We also asked management for administrative aide positions to relieve RNs of non-nursing activities that remained after all the other support services had assumed their functions. We found that these non-nurses could quite capably handle two to four units each. We have a total of twelve, one of whom serves as dispatcher for the active escort section of our service. Table 1 compares the traditional staffing plan and our present organization.

(At the time of this presentation [1978] we had forty-nine LVNs on duty. They were employed in certain specified areas to determine whether there were enough functions not requiring an RN to justify that staff category in our primary nursing organization. The LVNs were assigned to the orthopedic surgical unit, an active medical unit, a rehabilitation unit, a nurse-administered unit, and the alcohol treatment unit. They were designated as associate nurses and worked directly with the RNs.

In September 1980, the LVNs were reduced by attrition to nineteen and are assigned only to the orthopedic, rehabilitation, and alcohol treatment units. This change was necessitated by the increasing complexity of nursing care required by our patients.

Table 1. Comparison of Traditional and Primary Nursing Staffing Levels and Costs

Service	Traditional Staffing Plan						Primary/Professional Nursing						
	Number of Units	RNs	LVN/NA	Other	Total	Salaries	Number of Units	RNs	LVNs	NA	Other	Total	Salaries
Medical	6	50	89	—	139	1,855,245	8	89	13	—	2.0	104.0	1,730,506
Surgical	5	51	78	—	129	1,752,345	6	92	14	—	2.6	108.6	1,803,125
Psychiatry	10	46	120	—	166	2,124,430	6	79	4	—	3.5	86.5	1,472,858
Special Care Units	3	44	41	—	85	1,223,775	4	67	—	—	1.4	68.4	1,193,982
Office, Chief Nurse including Nursing Ed.		19	—	4	23	460,856		15	—	3.4	6	24	425,711
Special Programs Other Assignment	8	39	36	—	75	1,078,380	14	49	25	—	2.9	76.9	1,166,608
Totals	32	249	364	4	617	8,495,031	38	391	56	3	18.4	468.4	7,792,790

The nursing assistants are assigned in escort activities and do not work directly with patients on the nursing units.

Our organization remains cost effective and attractive to RNs who want to "nurse." The management of our hospital continues to hold us accountable, both financially and for high quality nursing care. In this day of nurse shortages, we do not have a shortage; daily we receive nationwide applications from nurses who have heard about our RN staffing organization and about the satisfactions experienced by patients, their families, and the nurses alike.)

The net result of all our changes is a dramatic drop in the number of persons required for nursing service—from an activation plan of 617 to the present 469—a decrease of 148.

The salary costs are clearly lower in spite of the substantially increased number of RNs employed. These are reliable figures; the nursing service at VAH San Antonio has been studied consistently since we started in October 1973. In addition to studies made by the fiscal officer at the hospital, we have had studies made by budget and fiscal representatives from our central office; nursing service's continuing self-evaluation studies; and several studies by Hospital Administration Master's Program Residents. One of the residents set up a study that included the general nursing units but excluded the specialty units. It showed an annual saving of $625,547. He then added the cost of housekeeping personnel and still found a favorable cost differential of $430,297. You have already reviewed Table 1, which reveals the results of our original plan, including staffing for a larger number of units and programs, we are still achieving a significant cost saving.

Our turnover rate compares favorably with the national VA average:

	RN	LVN/LPN	NA
Nationwide	22.1%	32.3%	24.7%
San Antonio	16.3%	22.2%	17.9%

The figures speak for themselves as to whether an RN staff costs more. These figures were based on salary cost alone—a better comparison would include such other factors as supporting services, training and continuing education costs for nonprofessional nursing staff, turnover rates, patient and family satisfaction, staff satisfaction, and staff flexibility. We believe such a comprehensive comparison would reveal even greater savings and better patient care.

Staffing with RNs

by P.W. Miller

In 1973 we opened L. W. Blake Hospital, a 150-bed community hospital, in Bradenton, Florida. The hospital has expanded to almost 300 beds for adult medical/surgical and critical care patients, and is also the nucleus of an eighty-acre Medical Park which will offer comprehensive health care at all levels. A hospital-based home care service was developed concurrently with the expansion to 300 beds as a first step in developing comprehensive services.

Although we opened the hospital using traditional team nursing with RN, LPN, and NA staff, we soon switched to primary nursing with one RN and one NA permanently assigned for each ten-bed district, days and evenings. Nights we assign two RNs and three NAs for forty patients.

The first step we took while eliminating team nursing to pave the way for future changes was decentralization of the nursing department. Decentralization is essential to keeping costs down while maintaining quality of direct patient care. The salary savings gained by eliminating middle management was used to convert to RN staff as LPNs left by attrition.

A salary savings program can be instituted to help with a full scale reorganization. In the planning phase the salary savings program can be set up so that as the nursing department is decentralized and budgeted positions are vacated, each salary saved goes into a special account for the cost center. Initially these savings would generally be nursing administration, but can be transferred to other cost centers. A typical Organization Chart is depicted in Figure 1.

The long-range plan employed to transfer the nursing department to an RN staff will be presented in this paper.

Figure 1.

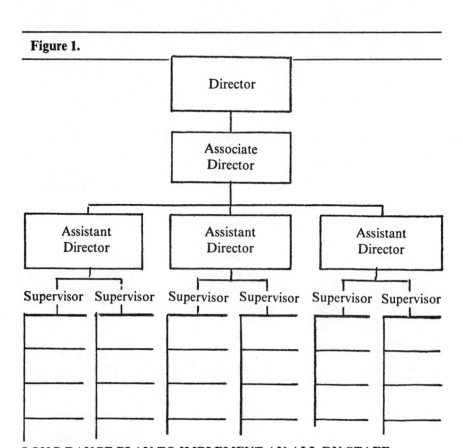

LONG-RANGE PLAN TO IMPLEMENT AN ALL-RN STAFF
First year

The best one or two supervisors should be retained to act as consultants to the head nurses, so they can develop fully into department heads. The "best" supervisors in this case are those not threatened by a helping role, who do not require tangible "status." Simultaneously, the actual duties of the day assistant director should be examined. Ask her to keep a diary of her daily activities, check her appointment book, and in short, ensure that she is doing valuable productive work, and also that enough meaningful work is delegated to her. If you find she is not fully occupied in productive work, restructure the role or eliminate it. Hagen and Wolf point out in their study of nursing leadership behavior that one poor personnel practice in the selection of supervisors was to appoint a person to the position of supervisor because she was difficult to get along with or had been employed for a long time. Often such persons get promoted to assistant director or director if they remain long enough in the institution. Nothing is sacred. Look at assistant and associate directors' *actual* day-to-day duties and activities as well as your own, if you are director of nursing. Many times we may fall into a pattern established before we were hired. Some common time-wasters are: daily rounds to patients' units, staff meetings for all RNs, attending all nursing department committee meetings, reading all daily reports from units.

During the first year the director should also get the new organizational chart on paper and approved. It is essential that the position of head nurse is officially at the level of department head.

Second Year

By the second year, head nurses are almost fully comfortable as department heads. They interview and hire their own employees, deal directly with department heads in other services, understand and participate in the budget process. The Director of Nursing must remember, however, that there should be systematic work on the supply and development of managers. It cannot be left to luck or chance. Assistant director/associate director roles have been studied and reorganized for increased productivity or are deleted. The two remaining supervisors who acted as consultants to the head nurse can now assume vacant head nurse positions or move laterally to staff positions.

Keep in mind the following points when designing managerial positions:

1. Staff to manage that is not too small. The staff should be large enough to challenge the growth of the individual as manager.

2. No "assistant to" staff positions. This is not a managerial function.

3. Career professional and manager means working boss.

4. Position carried out by one person with designated responsibilities.

5. Fancy titles are no substitute for rank and responsibility.

6. Any position that defeats one good candidate after aonother should be restructured.

Depending on the size of your hospital, you should decide if you need assistant or associate nurses. I find it quite easy to handle the following organization: the key to this is that once the individuals are all reasonably secure and functioning well in their own area, the only things that present difficulties are long-range planning for changes, incidents, and so forth. A monthly meeting is scheduled with each department head and director of nursing. These are scheduled for one hour but can be brief, if no problems exist. If planning or program changes are being done the full hour may be used. Between meetings each department head knows that he or she has access to the director of nursing at any time if it is essential.

In order to implement an orderly change to primary nursing with a staff of RNs and NAs, we had to phase out LPNs. This was perhaps our most difficult problem in implementation. When the idea was first discussed the local LPN school and association were very distressed. Since we are a developing health-care system offering several levels of care, we were able to offer "displaced" LPNs jobs in our extended care center and Rapid Patient Response system, a centralized patient call system. Many of our LPNs also entered the local RN program and are now ready to graduate as RNs. New units did not hire LPNs. As LPNs leave the other units, they are replaced with either an RN or NA. Although we have not completely phased out all LPNs through attrition, several units have accomplished this.

Third Year

By the third year the system moves from one RN and NA per ten-patient district to one RN per seven patients and four unit assistants per forty-bed unit. Although the nurse aide does not have any patient care assignment now, we found peaks and lulls in unit activity that could be met better by broadening the job description of nurse aide and housekeeping aide to unit assistant. This move will involve cross-training for both groups and ultimately reduce FTEs per day: from four NAs and two housekeeping aides to a total of four unit assistants with expanded job responsibilities.

Use of the four-day ten-hour-per-day work week with part-time shifts from 8a.m.–1p.m. and a fully part-time evening shift from 5–11p.m. also adds greatly to keeping costs down. The schedule is cyclic and repeats every two weeks:

```
S   M   T   W   T   F   S   S   M   T   W   T   F   S
—   on  on  —   —   on  on  on  —   on  on  on  —   —
```

Days	8:00– 6:00
Evenings	5:30–11:00
Nights	10:30– 8:30

A full-time (four-day) employee can be covered by a part-time (three-day) employee. All employees evenings are part-time except designated charge nurses who relieve the head nurse. Both head nurses and charge nurses work Monday through Friday on eight-hour shifts.

The question of cost and quality is one most people raise immediately when talking of an ALL-RN staff. The HAS report as shown in Table 1 can be used to show that, as the percentage of RNs increases, the salary expense stays the same or decreases.

The continuity of care is improved. Intrastaff communication regarding patient care has been simplified. Patients do identify "my nurse." Patients being readmitted ask to return to "2-North District-Mrs. Smith." Physicians have grasped the idea in most units and seek the primary nurse. If they still seek the head nurse only, she redirects them to the primary nurse.

Table 1.
Salary Expenses Stabilize or Decrease as the Percentage of RNs Increase.

December 1977

	LWB	National	State	Group
% RN	42.56	36.48	34.44	31.58
M/S Man-Hours	6.11	6.05	6.48	6.48
Salary Expense	25.67	28.62	27.54	27.54

With Primary Nursing We Have It All Together*

by Alice L. Dahlen

The nurses and patients at Meridian Park Hospital believe that the nursing staff truly has it all together. The basic reason is that registered nurses deliver all the primary nursing care. The nursing staff consists of registered nurses only, with the exception of two technicians in the operating room. The hospital also employs medical service technicians (ten full-time equivalents) who assist members of all departments, including nursing.

The chief reasons for using an ALL-RN staff were based on personal experience and nurses' expressed desire to deliver high-quality nursing care. We wanted to practice what we all believed, that the patient and his family are number one—not the technicians, nurses, or physicians.

The primary nursing care concept demands closer contact with patients and their families, allowing for more accurate assessment. The nurse at the bedside can see, feel and hear any changes and can react appropriately and directly. With no ancillary personnel to supervise, nurses are freed for patient care, which greatly enhances their satisfaction and patients' satisfaction.

By using only RNs, we theorized, we could use fewer personnel, thus diminishing communication errors and improving continuity of care. Patients, we hoped, would feel that their care was more individualized, because they would be relating to fewer persons.

This theory has been translated into practice. Primary nursing, to thrive, needs support from the environment. At Meridian Park Hospital, it has such support. Even though systems vary from hospital to hospital, taking a look at the systems that support primary nursing here is worthwhile.

THE SETTING

Our setting is an acute care facility of ninety-nine beds, which was opened in 1973. The basic design consists of two separate areas—one building houses all

---

the ancillary services, and the other area is the nursing towers. There are two nursing towers of three floors each. The building design anticipates any needed additions. These towers are connected with a short hallway and central core with utility rooms, examination rooms, and extra bathrooms. Each floor has two nursing units, each with seventeen single rooms with bath, clustered around the open nursing station.

We have approximately fifty nurses working full time and fifty who work part time to replace the full-time nurses during days off, sick leave, and vacation. This number includes the nurse clinician (head nurse), general staff nurses, and nurses covering the critical care unit. The basic staffing on a seventeen-bed medical/surgical nursing unit is as follows:

- 2 RNs - 7:00A.M. to 3:00P.M.
- 2 RNs - 3:00P.M. to 11:00P.M.
- 1 RN - 9:30A.M. to 6:00P.M.
- 1 RN - 11:00P.M. to 7:00A.M.
- 1 RN - 11:00P.M. to 7:00A.M. as a float between the two units on a floor
- 1 nurse clinician I covers both units, works 40 hours/week, and is included in the nursing hours for that floor.

Five of the six units house medical, surgical, and orthopedic patients. The sixth, the critical care unit, has six beds for intensive care/coronary care and eight beds in the special care unit.

Carpeting, primary colors, and wood paneling give a cheerful feeling. The hospital was designed to use Herman Miller Action Office for the nurses' station and offices. This is a system using modular components that are interchangeable, colorful, and durable. The pieces can be put together as needed and easily changed when the need changes. The walls, drawers, file cabinets, and shelves are portable. The equipment is beautifully adapted to an automatic restocking system.

A supportive attitude, from the board and administration through the whole staff, allows all members to work in a relaxed professional atmosphere. The philosophy is to let the professionals do their work without too much supervision, but when help is needed, all nursing personnel, regardless of position, are expected to pitch in.

The selection of nurses is important to the success of an ALL-RN program. Each applicant is first interviewed by the assistant director of nursing service, who explains the basic functioning of the hospital and determines if the nurse qualifies for employment, based on education, experience, motivation, and the desire to deliver total nursing care. The educational preparation of nurses on Meridian's staff varies from a master's degree in nursing to an associate degree.

After the initial interview, the nurse clinician (head nurse) for the designated area conducts the final interview and gives consent for hiring.

Hiring only persons attuned to bedside care is crucial. Few nurses here have resigned because they did not enjoy primary nursing care, and staff morale is high. Many have said there is less friction here between nursing personnel than in the places where they were previously employed.

New systems and forms were designed to facilitate primary nursing. One system that demands little of the nurse is restocking supplies. After the nurses have determined the quantity of supplies for their units, the medical service technicians maintain that level. These employees assist all departments by transporting patients and delivering supplies, clean and soiled. In nursing, they assist in weighing bed patients, male catheterizations and perineal care when necessary, and traction setup.

Another helpful system is the pharmacy nurse. Pharmacy is very much a part of patient care at Meridian Park Hospital. The pharmacy keeps a patient profile that lists all the medications the patient was taking prior to admission, plus those currently prescribed. Pharmacy nurses, working out of the pharmacy twenty-four hours a day (two on the day, two on the evening, and one on the night shift) give all routine medication and mix and start all intravenous solutions and blood. They work closely with the pharmacist and the unit nurses.

The unit nurses administer the prn and stat medications only. Before administering any medications, the pharmacy nurses check patients' charts for new orders, discontinuation of medications, and notations on side effects. The ICU/CCU area is the exception to this system. Critical care nurses administer all drugs and IV solutions to their patients.

Recently, local college students compared our pharmacy system with two other systems used in hospitals. Their findings indicated that errors in our system usually happened as one of a kind, not repetitively as in the comparison institutions.

One system we discontinued is the nursing visible card file. The nurses use patients' charts as do the physicians for reading and recording the patients' progress and for checking medications.

To organize their work, the nurses designed a worksheet that covers a twenty-four hour period and is kept at the nurses' station. This assists in the continuity of care by showing X-ray and lab orders, intravenous solutions, and so forth. To keep progress notes free from routine nursing measures, we placed a checklist on the back of the graphic sheet in the chart, so the nurses need only check for such comfort and hygiene measures as backrub and shampoo. The form has space for recording the patient's activities of the day, specimens sent to the lab, and so forth.

We found that the visible card file had become a crutch to most nurses, and we believed that the less we rewrote orders in different places, the less the possibility of error. To increase continuity, the nurses make rounds with each other at the change of shifts. Oncoming nurses are introduced to the new patients, and patients are included in planning their care for the next eight hours. Several patients have told me how much they appreciate this.

One of the most important systems we decided to use, I believe, is the problem-oriented record. The admitting personnel make up the basic chart and take both patient and chart to the assigned nursing unit.

The physicians initiate the problem sheets and all personnel—physicians, nurses, respiratory therapists, physical therapists, dietery workers, and others—write observations on the progress notes. This means that the nursing care plan is no longer on a visible card file where only nursing personnel see it but is a permanent part of the patient's chart for all to see.

The nurses are pleased with the problem-oriented system. They believe the physicians are now reading what they write and that what they write is worthwhile information. POMR charting is briefer, but certainly not easier, as it requires one to think and organize one's thoughts before recording. The POMR offers another satisfaction: the opportunity to document patient outcomes and nursing conclusions about problems.

The key form that cuts paperwork for the nurses is our physician order form. This form has six colored sheets. The first sheet remains on the chart, and the other five sheets (the carbon copies) are serrated so that they can be torn off. These sheets are sent to each of the following departments: laboratory, X-ray, dietary, and pharmacy. The remaining sheet may go to EEG/ECG, respiratory therapy, or physical therapy.

On receipt of orders, staff in each department perform requested activities. Having order sheets gives each department staff an idea of what is happening to the patient as a total person and relieves nurses of the secretarial duties that many nurses performed in the past. Each department is responsible for placing reports of laboratory tests, X-rays, operations, and so forth on the patients' charts.

COSTS AND MONITORING

One crucial item to consider when contemplating the ALL-RN concept is cost. The room rate at Meridian Park Hospital is in the same range as the two-bed rate in the Portland metropolitan area, of which we are a part. Our nursing care hours (hours of nursing for each patient for a twenty-four hour period) are usually around 4.0, while most hospitals in the area run 4.9 to 6.5 or higher. In the fall of 1977, in contrasting cost estimates for an ALL-RN staff with two more traditional staffing patterns, I found our costs were less. One of the hospitals in the study used RNs, LPNs, aides, and ward clerks. The other hospital used RNs, LPNs, and ward clerks, but no nurse's aides.

I used 4.0 nursing care hours for our hospital, and 5.6 nursing care hours for the other hospitals. I included the pharmacy nurses in our cost and IV nurses in theirs, trying to match the three hospitals as closely as possible. In the hospital that used all levels of staffing including aides, the cost per month to operate the nursing department for thirty-four beds (or two 17-bed units) came to approximately $27,573. For the other hospital, the cost estimate amounted to $28,407. For Meridian Park Hospital, the cost estimate was $25,288.

To determine the meaning of the words, "high-quality nursing care," a definition was needed, along with standards for delivering care. These standards, written when the hospital was opened, are reviewed by the nurses yearly and changed as needed. Nursing care, as documented on the patient charts, is reviewed monthly for quality. The monitoring process is also indispensable for determining staff educational needs.

Definite and clear position descriptions, written at the beginning, are modified periodically. Nursing is now at a point where evaluations must represent an honest review of job performance, as judged by patient chart review.

MONITORING QUALITY

The nurses also evaluate each other while they work together. Nurses now look upon evaluation as a tool for growth, with evaluation having a positive rather than punitive focus. For example, a nurse on the day shift thought that one evening nurse was not performing at the level she could or should be. The two nurses on days recommended that the evening nurse trade shifts with one of them for a month. The day nurse then shared her skills with the evening nurse to help her grow.

At the time of evaluation, each nurse is expected to write goals and objectives for herself for the coming year. These goals, in turn, feed into the yearly departmental goals.

So how do the nurses at Meridian Park Hospital spend their time? First, they do the many routine nursing tasks—vital signs, hygiene services, dressing changes, and irritations. They listen to patients and assist them and their families to meet pressing psychosocial needs. From my observation, nurses do better than anyone else at responding to their patients' psychosocial needs.

The nurses are also much involved in teaching patients and families— preoperative and postoperative sessions, and instructions about various tests. They have established ongoing classes for patients and families regarding postcoronary care and care of diabetes.

Does RN Staffing Escalate Medical Care Costs?

by Jean Forseth

"We can't do primary nursing here; it costs too much." Nursing staff, physicians, and heads of departments reacted this way when the change to an ALL-RN staff was discussed. In 1975, our concept of primary nursing developed. For us, it has had a two-fold definition: individual nurse accountability and an essentially all-professional staff. Because of the staffing pattern, costs were greatly feared. This study involved a 200-bed acute-care general hospital without physician house staff or medical training programs. Although there are limitations, the findings demonstrate comparable or lower cost in the unit with ALL-RN staffing.

Bayfront Medical Center in St. Petersburg, Florida, found the change to primary nursing had a positive effect on bed occupancy levels, staffing, turnover, nursing morale and, cost effectiveness[1]. Ciske also found decreased turnover rate for RNs and LPNs[2]. A study at Evanston Hospital demonstrated a change to primary nursing. The system was "not more expensive than team nursing if the first-line staff is clinically competent and fiscally accountable." HAS reports were the data base for that study. Quality of care measures were highly favorable to primary nursing[3]. Engineering studies in North and South Carolina showed that on the average, aides are utilized only 65 percent of the time, the LPNs 95 percent of the time, while the RN was utilized 100 percent of the time. Clark used these findings to demonstrate that those differences can result in the aide *costing* the hospital 8¢ more an hour than the RN[4].

Despite the number of articles referring to high quality of patient care in primary nursing, I am asked for the data on costs of the unit twice as often as quality measures. Like it or not, cost sways most decisions. Does primary nursing really cost more?

Experience with developing our concept of primary nursing convinced me that there is nothing inherent in the primary nurse role that can increase unit costs. Some units named "primary" use the concepts of responsibility and

Table 1.   Comparison of Nursing Unit Staffing Patterns

| # of Beds | DAILY STAFFING | | | Total Full-time Employees |
	DAY	EVENING	NIGHT	
	3 North—Primary Nursing Unit			
28	5 RNs	5 RNs	2 RNs	22
	1 clerk	1 clerk	1 LPN	
	3 South—Team Nursing Unit			
36	3 RNs	3 RNs	2 RNs	34,6
	2 LPNs	2 LPNs	1 LPN	
	5 aides	3 aides	1 aide	
	1 clerk	1 clerk	—	
	4 North—Team Nursing Unit in Transition to Primary Nursing			
35	4 RNs	3 RNs	3 RNs	34.2
	1 LPN	2 LPNs	1 LPN	
	4 aides	2 aides	—	
	1 clerk	1 clerk	—	
	4 South—Team Nursing Unit			
36	3 RNs	3 RNs	1 RN	34.6
	1 LPN	1 LPN	1 LPN	
	6 aides	4 aides	1 LPN	
	1 clerk	1 clerk	2 aides	

Note: 1 head nurse included in full-time employee total but not in daily staffing figures.

accountability, but do little or nothing to upgrade their quality of care by staffing predominantly with RNs. Changing the staffing mix most affects costs because salary differences make up the major portion of a unit's budget. Overtime has been mentioned as higher by some but has not been our experience[5].

STUDY DESIGN

Table 1 shows staffing patterns for four nursing units. Three North, a primary nursing unit, receives many patients in transfer from ICU/CCU. Designated for medical rehabilitation, cancer and myocardial infarction are most common diagnoses. Three South, a team nursing unit, is a general medical unit with eight private rooms equipped for isolation patients. Four North, a team nursing in transition to primary nursing, is a general surgery ward that receives all open heart surgicals within two days of surgery if uncomplicated. Four South, a team nursing unit, is designated for orthopedics and neurosurgical patients. It services a high portion of patients needing rehabilitation.

Each team nursing unit's full-time employees and staffing pattern includes one LPN on the day and evening shifts who is presently budgeted out of pharmacy and whose duties are medication administration on the unit. Since medication administration is usually provided in nursing service budgets and the primary nursing unit does not need these LPNs, their salaries and hours have been added to the team units. The hospital temporarily lays off on a rotating basis nursing personnel who are not needed when the daily occupancy drops below 85 percent. Thus, costs are controlled on a day-to-day basis by each head nurse.

The major question is whether salary expense per patient day is higher in the primary unit using almost ALL-RN staffing than in the units with more nonprofessional nursing staff. There are many variables which must be considered. In order to compare salary by patient day, the patient days should be held constant to watch how the salary cost varies. Since patient days are made up of number of beds, how many of those beds are occupied, and the number of days in a month, any variation in those items can widely distort the results. Attempts have been made in this study to adjust for the uncontrollable differences in bed capacity and occupancy from unit to unit. I have found that even a decrease of one bed between units causes false high values in cost per patient day since the divisor is correspondingly small.

Level of care required by patients dictates staffing patterns and salary costs. Day-to-day adjustments in staff for patient acuity is not a completed program in our hospital. For the purpose of this study our rating scale has been divided into two categories: high and low. All units consistently have 60 percent of their patients in the high acuity category. When units are compared with each other, acuity on the primary nursing unit is rated 3-5 percent lower than on other units. In my opinion, nurses doing total patient care rank acuity lower than those doing part-task care. It would require an independent audit of our ratings to demonstrate that hypothesis.

Another major variable mentioned in several studies[6] is whether lower salary costs for the primary nursing unit can be explained by differences in pay rate. A new modality may tend to have higher percentages of new graduates than experienced nurses. Our unit has been functioning for almost three years. Since our salary scale is spread over three year increments, this variable is thought not to be a factor in this study. Midpoints in our salary scale are as follows: RN $6.36, LPN $4.36, and aide $3.19. Tables 2 and 3 show percentage of RNs on each unit at maximum pay level and comparison of the unit's total hourly pay rates.

Table 2. Percentage of RNs at Maximum Wage

3 North	(Primary)	48%
3 South	(Team)	53%
4 North	(Trans. Team)	45%
4 South	(Team)	62%

Because the mix of staff nurses, LPNs, and aides is our only concern in answering the question of cost, the salary level and hours of the head nurse and ward clerks have been deleted in Table 5. Cost figures with head nurse and ward clerk and without them will be shown for the sake of clarity (see Tables 4 and 5). Conclusions are based on figures without head nurse and ward clerk to show as pure a comparison as possible.

DATA COLLECTION

The study period available was limited by a change in capacity from twenty-two to twenty-eight on 3 North in November, 1977. Actual total salary and wages paid for each unit from December, 1977 through March, 1978 were used as a basis for salary per bed determination. Productive hours for the study include all regular hours, overtime, orientation time, and head-nurse hours. Nonproductive hours include holiday, vacation, and sick time. This division of categories was predetermined by our accounting system. Patient days are computed by adding the census of each day to determine a monthly sum. Actual head nurse and ward clerk wages and hours were used for subtraction. Total pharmacy medication LPN salaries and hours were divided by four (the number of units in the hospital using that system) and applied equally to the three units in the study.

Table 3. Unit Hourly Pay Rate

	With HN & WC	Without HN & WC
3 North (Primary)	$6.26	$6.46
3 South (Team)	$4.79	$4.85
4 North (Trans. Team)	$5.13	$5.15
4 South (Team)	$4.67	$4.67

As mentioned earlier, lower bed capacity and/or occupancy increases the cost per patient day. In an effort to equalize the differences apparent between our study units, 3 North was projected to thirty-six bed size by adding salary cost and hours for one additional RN each shift using $6.46 as expected salary rate. Twenty-eight bed figures are shown to illustrate the inability to compare two units of differing bed capacity.

Table 4
Four-month Average Comparison Figures for All Staff of All Units

	Primary		Team		
	3N-28 beds	3N-36 beds	3S-36 beds	4N-35 beds	4S-36 beds
Occupancy	87%	87%	84%	85%	83%
Salary & Wages	24,557	29,253	28,869	30,709	28,456
Productive Hours	3,662	4,389	5,623	5,500	5,483
Nonproductive Hours	288	304	395	490	610
Patient Days	739	950	908	900	906
Salary Expenses Per Patient Day	33.23	30.79	31.79	34.12	31.41
Total Hours Per Patient Day	5.35	4.94	6.63	6.66	6.73

Table 5
Four-month Average Comparison Figures for All Staff of All Units
Excluding Head Nurses and Ward Clerks

	Primary		Team		
	3N-28 beds	3N-36 beds	3S-36 beds	4N-35 beds	4S-36 beds
Occupancy	87%	87%	84%	85%	83%
Salary & Wages	21,363	26,059	26,094	28,095	25,469
Productive Hours	3,050	3,777	4,995	5,021	4,910
Nonproductive Hours	257	273	381	432	541
Patient Days	739	950	908	900	906
Salary Expense Per Patient Day	28.91	27.43	28.74	31.22	28.11
Total Hours Per Patient Day	4.47	4.26	5.92	6.06	6.02

The figures reflect that the 3 North occupancy rate is 3 percent higher than that of the other units. If the other unit's patient days were applied to 3 North, and salary and hours correspondingly reduced, the primary nursing unit costs are equal to or less than the other units.

Every effort has been made to ensure accuracy of the results. Accounting journal entries, unit monthly budget justification reports, and number of vacant positions were used to verify accuracy. In review of the schedule sheets it was apparent that both 3 South and 4 South frequently had vacant positions. This was not true of 3 North and 4 North which had almost all positions filled every day as need indicated by census. Had all positions been filled on the team units, their salaries would increase by $500-$1000 per month. If fully staffed, 3 South and 4 South cost increases by over 50¢ per patient day.

Other variables inherent in such a study are sick time, overtime, and turnover. All staff except RNs are on an Earned Time System of benefits. All nonproductive time becomes one category, "vacation." Thus, if sick time is lower or higher in RN than aide staff, it cannot be determined. RN overtime was compared from unit to unit. Twenty-four RNs on 3 North had four month average overtime of twenty-nine hours per month. The team units with fourteen to sixteen RNs averaged twenty-five hours per month overtime. Nonprofessional staff have little overtime in our hospital. Turnover of all nursing staff on each unit for the year 1977 is shown inTable 6.

Table 6

Annual Turnover Rate of All Nursing Staff in All Units During 1977
3N (Primary) 23%
3S (Team) 37%
4N (Trans. Team) 29.3%
4S (Team) 25%

Note: Temporary vacation relief eliminated from computations.

A similar six-month study of cost per patient day in 1976 with the primary unit at twenty-two beds (adjusted to thirty-six beds) showed essentially the same results as in Table 5. At that time no staff accrued earned time. Comparisons of the units for other variables showed much lower sick time and turnover costs in the primary nursing unit.

CONCLUSIONS AND RECOMMENDATIONS

The data from this study confirm that if costs are controlled, primary nursing does not escalate medical care costs. Any system not held accountable can waste the money of patients and taxpayers. As primary nursing quality measures are shown to be high, decisions to change to primary nursing should be based on need for upgrading the patient care in a department. Local availability of nurses may limit the number of nurses possible in a staffing pattern. Cost factors, however, should not be feared.

For the purposes of further studies, we recommend that units of the same bed capacity, occupancy, and possibly dual leadership be utilized. Interinstitutional studies are recommended. These studies must include careful definition of terminology. For instance, few institutions mean the same thing when speaking of what is included in hours of care. Quality studies must continue as better instruments for quality measurement are developed.

In summary, we have found ALL-RN staffing to be a feasible and worthwhile change. From a purely economic standpoint, the change can be justified.

REFERENCES

1. Isler, C. Rx for a sick hospital: Primary nursing care. *RN,* February, 1976, pp. 60-65.
2. Ciske, K.L., Primary nursing: An organization that promotes professional practice. *Journal of Nursing Administration,* January-February, 1974, p. 28.
3. Corpuz, T. Primary nursing meets needs, expectations of patients and staff. *Hospitals,* June 1, 1977, 51, 95-100.
4. Clark, E.L. A model of nurse staffing for effective patient care. *Journal of Nursing Administration,* February, 1977, p. 22.
5. Marram, G. Flynn, K., Abaravich, W., and Carey, S. *Cost Effectiveness of Primary and Team Nursing.* Wakefield, Massachusetts: Contemporary Publishing, 1976.

Reports of the ALL-RN Nursing Strategy Development Discussion Groups

by Genrose Alfano, Marguerite Burt, Luther Christman, Barbara Brown, Sylvia Carlson, June Werner, Margaret McClure, and Barbara Donaho

Alfano: To present the conclusions and recommendations regarding the challenges and obstacles identified yesterday, we will maintain the same order of speakers. I'll ask Marguerite Burt if she will share her group's summary with us.

Burt: We concluded that it is most important to learn the nursing process and our strategies are accordingly categorized in keeping with this process.

Under the category of administrative educational planning we propose the following:

1. Development of a knowledge base prior to proposing a particular method of practice as the solution to better patient care.

2. Development of a common language before initiating action on the proposal.

3. Identification of the educational needs of every one affected by a change in nursing practice, the support services as well as top management.

4. Assurance of commitment to change at each level in nursing and in continuing education. One way to ensure that our efforts meet with success is establishing a well-coordinated inservice or educational program on the nursing process, interpersonal skills, nursing assessment skills, and interviewing techniques. We want strong clinical instructors, strong nurses at each level, and a strong nursing education faculty that can arm us with the knowledge needed for change.

5. Recruitment of a nurse researcher employed by the individual health-care facility (or shared with other hospitals, if necessary) to study the development of a proposal, to identify variables and problems, to select appropriate tools.

Under the category of implementation, we suggest:

1. Primary nursing. If your hospital has not changed to primary nursing, get it under way. Stop worrying about semantics and look instead at commitment, accountability, and so on. Initiate a pilot program and make sure it has the resources to be successful. Identify the interested nurses. Ask them to compete for assignment in the pilot unit and earn the right to be primary nurses. One of the primary nurses in our group remarked that for six months now she has been in a pilot program in which all the nurses vied for positions. They are titled associate nurses; at the end of six months, they hope to be awarded a primary nursing certificate. We liked that idea very much. We think that the nurses who are involved at the direct patient-care level should be challenged to develop the defined expectations, to change to meet the performance standards and develop the expected roles.

2. Encourage publication of our plans and communicate role models to all concerned. Identify role models by looking at the practitioner who is giving that care, who influences others, and recruits others to be those role models.

3. Encourage nursing rounds, not only on the pilot unit by nurses themselves between shifts but between units and by other people in surrounding hospitals.

The category that we spent the most time discussing was political strategies, which we believe are an absolute necessity.

1. If we are going to face the increased cost of health care, we must assemble facts about costs and benefits.

2. We must publish with much greater frequency positive findings about costs and benefits.

3. We must develop positive approaches to upward mobility programs for qualified nonprofessionals.

4. We must move aggressively toward closer collaborative relationships between nursing education and nursing service. While that has been said for one-hundred years, we believe that one way to close this gap now is to utilize the primary nurse in direct care.

5. We must communicate with our representatives in Congress concerning the need for increased enrollment in better baccalaureate schools of nursing, the importance of upward mobility, and the enhancement of those schools through well-qualified faculty. We must stress the need to provide opportunities to others in nursing who occupy crucial positions and yet are unable to function at the level of the professional nurse. We call your attention to the increasing numbers of LPN schools, the problems of staffing any school with well-qualified faculties. These programs dilute the practice of nursing.

6. We must pressure JCAH to write standards that require provision of direct care by RNs. Push by any means you have available, the appointment of an RN at the policy making level of JCAH. We encourage all directors of

nursing to discuss primary nursing, its costs and benefits with the RN repres
enting JCAH during their site visits.

The positive facts about costs can't be underestimated. Developing professional nursing elements in quality assurance programs, both within nursing
and medical audit, with a multidisciplinary approach should be required of us
all.

Finally, we turned to the issue of upward mobility. We talk about the
preparation of the professional nurse, but eventually some of us must be
guided toward certain decisions and so we challenge you, as chief nurse
executives, to stop providing clinical practice facilities for LPN and nursing
assistant training programs.

Alfano: At the summit conference in New York State when the 1985
resolution was being worked out, some of us wanted to challenge those
registered nurses who help to educate nursing assistants and LPNs to replace
registered nurses; however, it got no further support. One point that I want to
address is JCAH Standards. The commission distributes drafts of its revi-
sions and standards to directors of nursing service, the Society for Nursing
Service Directors, AHA, and other groups involved in setting standards.
How many directors of nursing service let the standards go through without
the ALL-RN provision because they do not have staff to implement on an RN
level? This issue must be faced. It is a question of whether administration and
leadership are ready to assume the risks.

Christman: Our group has a series of recommendations similar to what we
have just heard. The first issue was consciousness raising. How do we develop
among the staff members a sense of professional accountability and an
uneasiness about the intrinsic value of tradition? It's the responsibility of top
management to raise the level of consciousness of the staff with existing
resources within the organization. There is an enormous amount of literature
available for circulation among the staff.

The second recommendation was the development of a knowledge base
through a staff development program. Individuals need clear guidelines
concerning goals and how to achieve them. Effectively communicating that
new clinical competence and shifting life-style and behavior patterns to
accommodate new organizational strategies are necessary goals.

Analysis of the entire political setting within a particular hospital or agency
was another recommendation. How do we pull the components together
toward synergy to bring about change? The expectations of all our departments must be renegotiated, reorganized. New expectations, both from others and for others to nurses must be managed effectively which demands
organizational and political strategies of considerable depth.

The fourth recommendation continues from the third; that is, the issue of nurses reversing their role as task specialists to full practitioners as with patient accountability. This assumes that new skills and competencies will be acquired to carry out and express that altered role.

The fifth recommendation generated a lot of discussion. It centered around the need for hospital administrators to generate new types of patient support services and to ensure that these respond to new demands created by the shift in nurse attention to activities in the clinical setting. Without adequate support services, the best efforts of nurses will be lost. I might add we have a strong ally in the medical staff because that's one of their chief complaints.

The concept of regular evaluation and data gathering was discussed in great detail. In order to develop a course of action, everyone needs the data, not just top management. Persons in the action arena giving direct care must also share in the information that has been gathered and must understand how to use the data to enhance their own practice and that of their unit.

We were concerned about nursing education. We believe that it is a responsibility of persons in direct patient care to impress educators with the need for new forms of nursing education, role induction, and role socialization so that students arrive in the clinical arena equipped to handle the reality of present-day nursing practice.

Brown: Our topic was traditional intercollegial relationships. The following story should illustrate the point. This is a story about a doctor who went to heaven, replete with white lab coat and stethoscope. This doctor felt he had saved enough lives to entitle him to go straight through the pearly gates. He approached St. Peter and said, "I've saved so many lives, I've done my service for humankind. I think I ought to go right in." St. Peter said "I'm sorry, sir, but there are many people waiting in line who have done their service too. Now you just go back there and wait in line." The doctor sat there and waited. Suddenly a bearded man walked in wearing a long white coat and carrying a stethoscope around his neck. He walked right through the pearly gates. The doctor went up to St. Peter and said, "Hey, how come that guy gets to go in and I'm still sitting back there?" St. Peter said, "Well, that's God playing doctor."

I think that story speaks to the nurses' traditional concept of intercollegial relationships with MDs. To begin the process of establishing a true intercollegial relationship, we started with the basic understandings of power, authority, and influence and some leadership concepts. We then moved to developing interpersonal power and organizational power by looking at some of those concepts. We concentrated on the basic attitudes required for collaborative communications relating to both nonverbal and verbal communication skills and organizational structural changes facilitating collegial relationships.

We then progressed to a discussion of solid strategies and obviously concentrated initially on the MD collaborative relationship. We must reroute communications so that all information does not travel to the physician in charge and communicate directly. Incumbent with this change in channels of communication is the need for the registered nurse to communicate in an articulate manner.

We must correct such myths as nurses rising for doctors entering the nursing station. We must follow through on every physician complaint and develop a feedback system to handle complaints. But don't get caught up in the semantics of words such as equal or colleague, feeling you have to be equal. As one member of our group commented, we want maximum collaboration: "I'm not 'equal' with a twenty-year-old house physician who has just come into the system, nor am I 'equal' to the chief of the section." I don't expect or need equality, but I do want to establish collaborative communication. To use another example, if I have a bleeding aneurysm, I want a doctor. If I'm paralyzed, I want a nurse. If the paralysis is likely to have some permanent residual, then I need a nurse. We must get beyond our hangup of equality in terms of decision making.

Another area in need of strategy is assuring clinical competence; that's how we will establish collaborative ralationships. We must be responsive to cultural and ethnic differences, recognizing that we can't force an issue when we are working with individual staff nurses and individual physicians. Staff nurses must gain respect of others through competency. We should do whatever we can in each setting to stop this doctor/nurse game playing. A book that was recommended by one member of our group was *The Woman Executive.*

One issue that grew out of this discussion was our tendency to avoid difficult situations. We must assume a positive attitude and confront difficult situations head on.

Organizational structure can facilitate better nurse/physician relationships. One point that we raised was whether the nurse director membership on the medical executive committee should be official and carry voting privileges. Regardless of status, however, the presence of the nurse administrator on such a committee facilitates active collaboration in the organizational structure. Other members of the nursing staff should also serve on medical staff committees and medical boards. We must ensure, however, that those nurses who represent us can be articulate on behalf of nursing. In other words, don't send a nurse with no knowledge of epidemiology to an infection control meeting.

Another recommendation was to include the physician in the selection of key personnel for clinical areas. This is not to suggest that the medical staff should be decision makers in hiring, but it is politically advantageous to seek medical input if we want collaborative relationships between those key people. This also gives the nurse under consideration an opportunity to meet the chief of the clinical division, with whom she may be working. Another person suggested that this practice might lead to reciprocal behavior by physicians; for example, if they're recruiting chiefs of sections in the medical center, the nurse administrators might be involved in that selection process too. So we begin to collaborate on how we will work together from an organizational standpoint. One nurse in our group sent minutes of nurse management meetings to the medical management meetings and soon started receiving the minutes of the medical management meetings.

We discussed the need for joint education of nurses and physicians. Case-Western Reserve was one example. Someone suggested just programming to facilitate communication—for example, joint educational programs between Ob/Gyn and clinical experts who teach new residents/interns. Have residents or interns participate in developing a critical-care course. Patient-care conference committees were another example of working together to find a positive solution to difficult patient problems.

Introduce yourself to each clinical chief of the medical staff in an effort to establish some perspective on each person's background. Get to know them as individuals. Discuss with the medical staff your rationale for bringing in a new clinical person in nursing. Share resumes and backgrounds to establish an experiential base. Send a memo to the medical staff for every new nursing appointment to engender their respect for the clinical judgment and background of nurses joining the organization. Present new ideas to the medical staff for their feedback before reaching decisions, even though the decision rests with nursing. Doing so implies that we are willing to listen and we appreciate feedback.

We moved from the nurse/physician relationship to nurse/nurse and other interdepartmental collegial relationships. These are some positive strategies that we devised in this area. Interdepartmental management seminars and leadership effectiveness training programs were offered as ways to bridge interdepartmental barriers and get people to begin working collegially. We must change our performance evaluations and the punative nature of assessment and look instead at positive reinforcement to encourage both interdepartmental and peer relationships within nursing. A participative evaluation system was offered that included job profiles, expansion of management by objectives to include clinical-based competencies, and establishment of self-objectives within nursing. Conducting open forums with evaluations in writing and conference meetings were other ideas for nurse/nurse relationships and other departmental relationships. One of the constants in our discussion was the need to develop skills in group work. Our staffs must feel comfortable in the arena of intercollegial relationships.

The director of nursing must be visible and it was stated that the director of nursing has a right to be a person and sometimes ought to let people know what the irritants are. One was, we don't like the nursing office to be referred to as "square footage". We're not square feet, we are persons and we want to be related to in that way.

One of the ways that we can be more visible to others is by making rounds every week. We talked about visibility with nursing staffs and some suggested occasional regularly scheduled night rounds by nurse administrators other than those scheduled on those shifts so that staff will come to know the administrators and can feel comfortable talking to them in work settings, in their own settings. about some of their concerns. We should encourage nurses to look to each other for consultation. For example, every three months one group member's hospital has a swap shop to share learning experiences gained over the three-month period. This has been going on for seven years in that organization. I think we should publish an article about it.

Education and travel support by institutions help remove barriers and facilitates collegial relationships within nursing. We talked about patients and their families and how we can transfer and discharge and form consultation teams that are interdisciplinary to facilitate the best relationships. In the final analysis, an overall relationship must include the patient and the family.

Carlson: We began our workshop with perhaps the most important institutional constraint on the practice of professional nursing, the nurse herself. That old adage "we have met the enemy and it is us," to which I grudgingly refer, must give us pause. Now, we should be accentuating the positive and devising means to improve that particular image, which is, we are our own worst enemy. The key question is how we view the problem. If we really believe in the concept of an ALL-RN staff, we need only ask how can we implement it? We need not wait for someone else to grant us permission.

Professionals, theoretically, do not need outside permission; they should be able to move from the inside out to interpret the mandate given them by their licensure and by the consumer. In this regard, we need to consider not what is the definition of a nurse, which has been thoroughly explored, but what is the definition of a nursing leader? I came across a definition of a nursing leader in the book, *Nursing Leadership, Process and Theory,* which said that nursing leadership is a process whereby a person who is a nurse affects the action of others in goal determination and achievement. We have tended to view leaders as those who have been conferred authority through title. To be a professional and to institute professionalism we must look to every nurse as a leader. I would like to repeat that definition, for I think it applies to everyone who is an RN from the director of nursing to the staff nurse. Nursing leadership is a process whereby a person who is a nurse—notice no adjective before or after—affects the goal actions of others in goal determination and achievement. If we take this definition as a given, everyone, every nurse, is a leader.

One of the problems in nursing is not the power that we have by our titles but powerlessness. I brought an article from the April 6, 1978, *New York Times* Op Ed page which has relevance to this discussion. The old ploy that power corrupts and absolute power corrupts absolutely received a new twist in this editorial. It suggested that it is the powerless in positions of responsibility that construct fiefdoms out of functions, coerce when they cannot persuade, and count the paperclips rather than encourage independent action. After all, the ultimate weapon of the powerless, theoretically those in power, is to hold everyone else back. Therefore, those who have theoretical power are powerless if they do not give the power away. In fact, you gain power by giving it and sharing it. You become, in essence, more powerful. Power held and not used deteriorates.

Some of the problems we have had in the bureaucratic system of nursing, which is our own enemy, is the old traditional power. It is the constraint upon the professional nurse who is the leader at the bedside. Another definition of leadership is having a goal and being able to lead other people to move toward that goal. One way to accomplish this is turning our table of organization upside down. Rather than the traditional pyramid, we view it in reverse: the director of nursing lies at the bottom and serves as the support system for the entire group at the top, the nursing staff who care for patients. We look at our staff as supporting us, but we exist to support our staff. Turning that around we find that the staff is then able to support the patients. Barbara Brown's comments about communication and working together is part of that picture.

When we say we cannot do something because someone in a leadership position is preventing us from doing it, we must then look at the underlying philosophies and determine whether change is possible within the existing constraints. Do we really need another's permission to institute the professional nursing model? Do we need the administrator if we say it's cost effective? Do we need the physician if we say we are improving the direct delivery of patient care? Would they know the difference? Must we seek permission even of one another within the group?

I'd like to share with you two examples of how one implements change and removes constraints. One is the most simple and most direct way; it requires absolutely no one's permission. Having presented a program on the pilot study of a professional nursing model, I lunched with one of the head nurses from a local hospital. She said to me, "You know, I initiated a pilot program even before I heard you speak." I said, "How did you do it?" She said, "Very simply. We have a traditional nursing system in our hospital. One nurse came from an institution where they were doing what they call primary nursing, professional nursing, and she said she would like to try it."

Here was a head nurse who was a leader. She heard what the person had to say and said, "That's fine. Why don't you take a group of patients and forego being a team leader to see how it goes." Then she found another nurse who was interested and they set up a certain districting area and they just did what comes naturally. It doesn't really take a PhD and expertise to achieve this degree of competency. It comes naturally if you're a nurse. The nurses on the other side of the unit grew interested in this experimental group and began to ask the head nurse whether they could do it. She said, "Why not." Her supervisor didn't know; theoretically directors of nursing didn't know. In a very short time she had installed a professional nursing model as she and her staff saw it, and made it work. Then she was able to move the hospital through the ripple effect; other people began to hear that everyone is satisfied, patients like it, and doctors didn't complain because their patients were happy. That's one way to do implement change very simply. That nurse was a leader; she gave her staff the power and permission to bring about change.

The other example is a little more autocratic. One head nurse, who heard me speak, told this story to the audience. Her model was very simple, having been an exNavy nurse. She called her staff together (a self-directed staff) and said this is how I want you to do nursing. No more functional assignments. I am districting. You're going to do this! She gave it by fiat and said, "I installed primary nursing overnight." As part of professionalism, one doesn't tell patients what to do, you're working with the patient's self-determination. You don't perform ten o'clock ostomy care because it is convenient for the staff. One does it at a time that is comfortable and convenient for the patient. "You know," she said, "I no longer went and told the patient, 'I am giving you your ostomy irritation.' Would you believe I went in and asked him when he would like to have it." So I knew that her authoritarian posture was just that. She really understood the principles, even though she acted out what appeared to be a different philosophy.

Another alternative is sitting together and working out whole programs, outlines, and philosophies to present to the physicians. I'm not saying that's wrong. I think that's good; there is nothing wrong in doing it either way. The point is, change can move in any direction. It depends on who's the mover and who's the leader. It should be free to move in any direction when one is going to plan a strategy and do it professionally. The end result, we have all heard, is nurse satisfaction, patient satisfaction, and physician satisfaction, because the patient is happy. The doctor does not like to hear "I never saw a nurse" or "the coffee was cold."

Another issue that we discussed was orientation. I am concerned when people talk about the need for internships, the need for teaching people and having three, four, and six months programs to prepare nurses. Why do we look at the deficits of nursing education and think that inservice must overcome these deficits? Are we really going to translate nursing theory into nursing practice? The new graduate wants to do this, it comes naturally. What do we think we're teaching them when we say we're going to give them long orientations on how to be a nurse? My own feeling is that the students we get from the baccalaureate programs know how to do primary nursing. They just need us to facilitate their doing it, not to teach them. They may need an orientation program, but they don't need us to teach them.

As time began to run out, I wanted to end our session on a note that would give us hope. I mentioned that I found an embroidered blouse that had turtles on it, which I purchased for a program because I thought it had some significance. I was going to use it as a prop. On the front it said, "behold the turtle;" on the arms was printed, "he only makes progress when he sticks his neck out."

Alfano: Analogies to other professions create problems if one thinks about the physician who practices medicine and the lawyer who practices law. We stop practicing once we begin performing. One of the dangers of analogies is that they just don't hold true all the way, and there is a possibility that we must be proud of saying we are nurses and nurses do have prestige. At least we believe they do, and I think that patients believe that nursing, interestingly enough, has prestige. Often prestige is not equated with nurses and it might be well for nurses to point out that nursing and nurses are equated, so that nurses then will have prestige.

One of my greatest aims is to see nursing respected to the degree that one can say, "I am a nurse", and the response is similar to that generated by "I am a doctor", because we have the same prestige value. That will happen when not everybody is considered competent to do nursing regardless of preparation.

Werner: We discussed a management structure based on the administration of a clinical department rather than a service department. Inherent in that model, and this is our strategy to develop an alternative, was sustained accountability for all leadership positions; that is, you would reconstruct a department so that everyone had twenty-four hour accountability for a piece of the patient population. You would never have a supervisor who was only accountable for what happened in an eight-hour period. The top priority in such a structure would be the clinical competence of everyone, of staff nurses and of the leadership group in the department of nursing. That implies some retooling because we haven't expected supervisors to be clinically competent. We expected them to mind the store and keep the ship on course, but we really haven't expected them to be clinically competent. That means in terms of continuing education that we must develop resourceful programs to retool people in their mid-career who we now expect to be clinically competent. I think that is possible, depending on how we do it; certainly, we must respect what they have brought to nursing and who they are.

Under a good management structure, an ALL-RN staff means fewer employees and consequently reduced costs; it also means a higher quality of care. The ultimate strategy is to convert our obsolete management structures to a contemporary model which meets the needs of patients in terms of safety and quality and responds to the cost containment program in the country. Unless we can do it cost effectively, sad to say, we can't do it. We must learn how to do it cost effectively, and within a structure developed by nurses, not by hospital administrators, not by physicians, but by nurses. Many nurses in this country are skilled in developing clinical management structures. I can tell you that once having done it, you will all become your own expert.

Our group was very pragmatic. They are experienced, seasoned people, and many are nursing administrators. Our strategies included some basic assumptions. The nursing administrator must be unequivocally committed to the goal—without her commitment, nothing will happen. If she is supporting change reluctantly, without total commitment, it won't happen.

Characteristically in nursing, what have we looked at? We have looked at directors of nursing and supervisors. Who has supervision, SUPERvision—nobody. What we need is an organization chart with the patient at the top. The pyramid that Sylvia Carlson talked about is the one to which we should address ourselves. With nursing administration holding up that department, facilitating the staff, and with supervisors facilitating head nurses and head nurses facilitating the staff. With an ALL-RN staff, fewer people are needed to facilitate care to that patient. We need to start thinking about supporting from the bottom rather than directing from the top.

I want a bumper sticker that reads *nursing administrators are not omnipotent.* The expectation in a sense is that we are omnipotent. I refer you to an article that I wrote on this topic in *Nursing Administration Quarterly,* the Fall 1976 issue on leadership. The nursing administrator must plan to be indispensable in terms of the goal of facilitating an ALL-RN staff, if that is her goal. Our strategy was to develop a plan by the nursing administrator with her associates for presentation to the institutional approval mechanism. Right through to the board. "Do whatever it takes to make it go in your institution"—I think that's very good advice.

There just aren't any recipes; you've got to map your own little piece of territory and determine how it would have to go there because you know, and if you don't know, you know how to find out. You may not like some of the answers. This should include a rationale in terms of the value system of the approval body. You've got to take into consideration as you put this together their prides, fears, and their preconceived notions, and develop the proposal on the basis of that value system. You've got to determine how to get it through. If their public image is terrifically important to them, push the public image. If they are inundated with law suits and worried about litigation, push safety. Write the proposal in terms of what you're up against. That's political savvy. You really must know the environment in which you work.

I question the validity of just doing it without telling anyone. Perhaps that would be the easier way in one sense, but if you're going to move to an ALL-RN staff, there's the business of paying them, of posting the position, of converting physicians. You must be in concert with your personnel department and it's great if you've got a good friend in that department. Negotiating to make the change workable is extremely important. We all assumed you would never do this without a pilot unit. You would just never go in and say, we're going to do this throughout the institution. You take one unit, a pilot unit, where success is predestined, where there is readiness on the part of the staff, where there is a payoff for patients in the program, where you have the feeling if you could convert to an ALL-RN staff, you could eliminate some of the problems or promote some of the things that the institution wants to promote. You've got to choose a unit on which there is some support from the physicians. Choose a unit where the physicians are amenable to reason.

Allow sufficient time before you begin to get baseline data on what you're doing now and then plan regular follow-up reports. You must have some baseline data, and you need the help of someone knowledgeable about data collection. There are myriad ways to get such assistance; one way, for example, is through your state university. Confer with the physicians who will be affected by the implementation of an ALL-RN staff. Request their input and ask their concerns about that unit. What would they like to see happen in a very open, honest way. Respond to their reasonable requests at every opportunity.

Showcase that unit for a Hawthorne effect. Get your public relations department in there. See to it that people know what's going on in that unit. Within reason, make sure that everyone knows you are exploring this system on a pilot unit. Develop a continuing education program for the unit based on that patient population and the method of assignment and nursing practice. Unless you built continuing education for the staff into the original proposal, it probably will not work. Our group talked about not knowing what the nursing process is and not knowing how to make people more competent in terms of nursing practice. There are many other aspects of continuing education, but you must build an ongoing program into that pilot unit.

We touched on the labor issue as an obstacle to overcome. We determined as a group that the department of nursing is vulnerable whether or not the staff is organized as far as a strike goes. We would plan for an ALL-RN staff knowing that there are no guarantees regarding labor problems. One member of the group who has a lot of experience in the area indicated that the nursing service administrator must thoroughly prepare to deal with an organized staff, including knowing how to prevent organizing, if possible. Failing that, the nursing administrator must prepare for the task of negotiating a contract and then using that contract to get what was needed in that institution wherever possible and not allowing the contract to impair safe patient care. If you are knowledgeable, it is possible to negotiate the contract to protect the patient—it's not easy.

We felt very strongly that we need to let it be known across the country that the Commission on Economic and General Welfare is supporting nurses who are demanding conditions that are contradictory to safe nursing care. We as nursing service administrators need to make that statement. There was absolute consensus in the group on that score.

We discussed agency nurses and said we certainly wouldn't want an ALL-RN staff comprised of a majority of agency nurses but we could see using them occasionally. There is some concern about the role of nursing service in nursing education. The necessity to build really good effective collegial relationships with others in your institution who are in education. We discussed the need to open up our institution so that faculty could become clinically competent in the areas in which they have students and our right to expect that all faculty working in our institutions be clinically competent. That takes some effort on our part. This is particularly imperative in intensive-care areas. We need to express, if we're going to do this, the expectations of nursing service in terms of students. Here are their role models, an ALL-RN staff. How will we socialize students in terms of an ALL-RN staff? Will they come out of school thinking that if we employ them to take care of patients, that they're being used as aides? How can we help them see that this is really professional practice and that nursing service has an obligation there. I think the key phrase yesterday from a group of people who have the capacity to develop an ALL-RN staff under reasonable conditions was "start small and think big."

McClure: Our topic was one that I think every group identified as a problem and that is, the inconsistent supply of professionally qualified nurses. We decided we needed to attack three pieces of this problem of supply to our institutions; obtaining further education for competent staff who need to increase their competencies; obtaining further education for incompetent staff who need to increase their competencies; and ensuring an adequate supply of new practitioners into our setting.

Some of the strategies that we discussed related to how directors of nursing worked in groups. I suggested that directors of nursing are not very good group workers. We do not very often get together with other directors of nursing—the VA being one possible exception—to get our act together so that we do think as a group, so that we make our positions and our needs known. Directors of nursing are very good about doing their own thing in their own institutions, but if you look around the country, there aren't many organized groups of nursing service directors who are taking positive action as an influential force.

That's a political problem. If you're going to be political, you discover that groups are stronger than individuals politically. We talked about influencing legislators if you're attempting to improve the state university system. For example, one individual indicated that there were inadequate opportunities for baccalaureate students and too few for associate degree students in her particular area. They had tried to reverse that trend and the legislature overruled them.

We also discussed the fact that we have not yet been very smart about operating in the back rooms, using less formal contracts and approaches. We recognize that others accomplish their aims in this way and we should learn the rules.

We discussed the need for nursing service to operate with and influence the decisions of educators. Someof us have tended to be passive. One woman in our group said, "Recently the university in our area decided to reduce the clinical experience in the hospital to thirteen days, two of which are orientation and evaluation." She complained that this limited clinical experience was inadequate for the entire senior year. Few people in the group disagreed with her. We considered the best strategies to handle such matters. Perhaps it's time for nursing service to visit the educators and ask "What do you think you're doing; who do you think you're preparing?" The people who go into community nursing need hospital-based nursing experience and most people who are in public-health settings want those they hire to have that experience.

Nursing service directors have the upper hand with educators and often don't realize it. Educators depend on nursing service directors for clinical facilities. It is a key to their survival, and we fail to recognize how very important that is to them. Because we hold that key, we can negotiate about what we would like to get versus what we're willing to give—trade-off on educational opportunities for staff; inviting their faculty to our in-service; allowing some of our people to go to some programs offered by the school. In other words, doing some of the trading that is possible if you recognize that you're in a position to negotiate and being more active than passive in relation to that.

We also discussed some of the strategies about which you might want to negotiate, for example, joint appointments and input into curriculum committees from individuals in nursing service. Those things that we think we could do jointly and do better. We talked also about the importance of counseling high school students into the right nursing programs so that people do not find themselves caught in an educational system that is inappropriate to the level of what they want to do. One woman from California indicated that in San Francisco, I think it is, students who go into any kind of nursing program must take a three session mini-course as a prerequisite in which they learn about the various kinds of nursing programs so that they can identify their own goals and decide which of the programs they should enter. Of course, my private opinion is that there shouldn't be so many options, but that's not a surprise to anyone.

When we talk about supply, we must talk about many things, including the people who are out there that we are trying to get. Barbara Brown alluded to the importance of a good recruitment program and we discussed some of the things that you would put into a recruitment program. Advertising in national magazines was discussed and it does keep one's name in the forefront so that if people decide to move to your area, they may think of your institution rather than another. Describe in national advertisements what you have to offer, both in your practice setting and your community, because sometimes that is attractive to people. As another recruitment device, it was suggested that individuals hire baccalaureate students for summer and weekend programs. Many of us are doing this and finding it an excellent recruitment device if it is a positive experience for the student. You must not only get them but ensure that all the right things happen for them. In states where continuing education is required by law, one individual indicated that the fact that her hospital had become an approved provider meant that RNs in that state could come to work at that hospital and get their mandatory continuing education hours free of charge. That was a very good recruiting device and it is something for us to think about.

We discussed the importance of nurses seeing a nurse rather than a personnel representative when they respond to employment opportunities. Everyone in our group decided that really is a very important item, although some of us have difficulty wrestling it from the personnel department. A dual career ladder within the institution was also suggested. Make it clear to people that they need not go up through the administrative ladder to be promoted but that they can be promoted along clinical lines. Many hospitals are doing this. We closed the recruitment issues by saying that the best recruitment device is a satisfied staff nurse who talks to her friends and I must tell you, that's the absolute truth.

We talked about how to get acceptance of primary nursing by nurses. This is what you must do. One hospital is instituting primary nursing unit by unit. If members of the unit don't want primary nursing, they're permitted to move to another unit. It's still unclear what will be done with the last few units which will be full of these people.

We talked about the acceptance of primary nursing by the non-nursing component. This is what's interesting. Barbara Brown told me at the break that her group noted my reactions to her report. They said I had several nonverbal responses. I was laughing at one point when Barbara Brown mentioned the importance of explaining to people in advance what you're planning to do. In our group what we said was, don't talk too much about what you're trying to do with people who are not directly involved. Do not go to the executive medical council ahead of time and talk about primary nursing because then they begin to give you all the reasons why you cannot and should not do it. Keep quiet about it, do it, and let them come and tell you how wonderful it is. We closed with the notion that the kind of changes we were talking about at this conference are going to take time. We all must recognize that and muster the patience to see it through.

Donaho: Our assigned topic was to look at the obstacle of established role definitions for nurses and supporting personnel. I assumed that the role definitions were established regardless of whether they appeared in writing or were ingrained in the institution, meaning that many of the staff have never seen their job definitions, but that is what they're doing and that's what we must deal with. We must deal with the process of changing the performance or the behaviors that we're observing. We spend no time talking about the difference in job descriptions and the items contained in the job descriptions. We assumed they were there, that's what the practice was, whether or not it was in writing.

I asked the group to identify the first step of the change process and where the responsibility and accountability rest. We identified the responsibility to plan and forecast for the organization that we're leading. We recognized that in planning and forecasting and, to use June's word, "SUPERvision," is very difficult to do. But without it we're going to slide around willy-nilly. Nobody will know our purpose for being, our direction. If we don't plan, you certainly cannot define the outcome you want. We clearly determined that the chief nursing officer, by whatever title, has the responsibility without exception to plan and forecast direction and to be heavily involved in all decisions about the "outcomes" to be pursued by nursing. Without this level of personal involvement, other forces and other people are very likely to stay with functional nursing, even if you prefer another direction.

Between planing and outcome is the time that we want involvement from the staff. We want their involvement in researching the literature, identifying the component parts of change which will enable them to develop new job descriptions, identifying the necessary attitudinal changes, and selecting the tools needed to produce change. Involve the staff in defining the resources involved and in determining preliminary cost projections, because then they will help control those costs.

As we considered all of these strategies, we finally recognized the enormity of the change process and that it will proceed slowly. It maybe subtle. You may be hard put to know that something is happening, unless you give yourself enough distance to step back and look at it objectively and identify your progress. The strategies that we can use for change were our focus and from there we moved our discussion to specific strategies. I broke the items discussed into two groups of strategies, according to my personal bias. The group just listed all the specific strategies and when I tried to separate them this morning, I broke them into categories.

The first strategy that I felt was essential was the need for nursing to understand the power base, particularly nursing leadership. We must identify the issues, know our support base, know our opposition. If we do not do our homework, we will walk into traps and experience setbacks.

Our second category was avoiding all or nothing situations when implementing change. You do not undertake a major change with a staff that is unequipped to handle it. At a given point, it's win/lose because you may have to compromise and move slowly or you slide back and forth and get concessions and change behavior and then keep building. Change doesn't happen by saying, "Tomorrow we're going to do this; you're all going to agree with me," and then you turn the page and it's there.

Plan and allow the staff some time and room for the change. Listen to their problems but don't jump to discard the change before it has had a chance to be assimilated. I've watched that happen. I've watched everyone get so grumbly and upset with a change that they said, "Oh, we have to go back," and then reverted. They've got to grumble. Good Lord, if they don't, they may not be alive! So allow time for that to happen. Develop a little "deafness" for the first part of change. It's a very wise strategy because you may respond to the wrong uproar and defeat something that you want accomplished.

Be prepared to support failure. Now that doesn't mean the whole project is lost. It means some little skirmish or some little part of change didn't go the way everyone thought it should. It means when you gave accountability to someone, she or he made a misjudgment. So they misjudged; help them learn from it and go on. Don't destroy the whole project because of one error and don't lose perspective because it's tempting and others will try to influence you. They'll say, "See, we told you it didn't work." You must be equipped to deal with those critics.

Be open and honest about change. You might want to time your openness and I agree with Maggie McClure that it is appropriate at times to have hidden agendas and it is appropriate at times to have some flags when you implement change. If you get caught, acknowledge it. I get caught in a lot of things and I kind of grin and say, okay, you got me. Be honest about it. Don't deny that you got caught or that you were trying a strategy that didn't work quite the way that you hoped it would.

Give credit where credit is due. I may well know exactly the direction in which I want things to go but if I've been successful in leading and giving the staff some choices and options, other staff members perceive that the idea came from the group; that's fine. I'll be glad to give them the credit for that. That helps create other ideas and suggests to the staff that you are listening. One other must is a provision for individual and group support systems during the change process. You must channel the feelings, frustrations, anger, and successes and challenge them so that they can be dealt with. If someone is angry and the only vehicle to release anger is one another, it can destroy incentive and creativity.

As I've gone through many of these change processes unit by unit in my setting I've used a highly skilled counselor who is comfortable in taking forced referrals because not everyone wants to learn the source of her or his anger. It's between them, I don't know anything about it, I don't need to know anything about it, I don't need to know what the conversations are; the counselor knows my overall department goals and she's been very successful in helping individuals decide that they really do want to be part of the change or acknowledge that they are in the wrong spot at the wrong time and should move out.

Don't feel badly when you lose some people, it may be the best thing that can happen to you and them. Using the group support system as a group, the staff can begin to learn to support one another and say, "I tried this and it did work for me," and begin to challenge each other, "Well, why in the world did you do it that way, why didn't you make the decision yourself." I can't overemphasize the necessity to use this strategy heavily. The staff needs it, the leadership needs it and we often forget that leadership needs it. We often spend time supporting the staff without recognizing that the leadership may also be taking a great deal of stress and strain. Another important strategy for implementing change is appointing a head nurse to the unit that is accepting of the change and is an identified change agent in a positive sense.

The other group of strategies that I would give to you is evaluation of the appropriateness of change for your setting. A pilot unit is a good idea but again, evaluate it; it depends on your size, and on your situation. Inherent in a pilot project is evaluation, some followup of the program. The group suggested that seeking and carefully selecting volunteers to staff the pilot unit is a very desirable thing. The use of a pilot director can be an advantage; it can also be a disadvantage, but look at it as a potential strategy. Outside consultants are another possibility; often unfortunately we are not prophets in our own land and it does help to bring in strangers. If you are going to bring them in, define for them what you want them to do, what they are there for, or you may find they've accomplished something that wasn't in your package of objectives. Outside agencies can be used to set standards, give some direction to the whole health-care system. Use them to your advantage if, again, it's appropriate.

Find ways to sell the idea. Begin to generate enthusiasm; get people to support and speak out in your organization. Sending staff to another hospital to see how other places have implemented change is sometimes a good approach. Getting them out to educational programs is another idea. It may reinforce the staff; it may help them see they're on the right track.

Our group spent a fair amount of time on the strategy of involving the troublemaker—identifying that individual who has been vocal. Evaluate this situation carefully to determine whether it's worth spending the time to train or groom them into supportive leadership. Most of the time troublemakers are already in a leadership role, the question is whether you can turn them around to the point where you want them so that they can help. I've often said to troublemakers when they've brought things to me of one magnitude or another, are they coming as the problem or with a problem. They know that I expect some possible solutions from them.

Another strategy is joint deliberations with other disciplines or departments. Again this can be appropriate for the setting depending on what part of that job function you plan to change. If you want to move a job into another department, joint deliberations are very effective. There's nothing that angers me more than another discipline coming to me and saying "You are going to do this and this is the deadline for doing it." I appreciate joint deliberations and they have their place, whether they are with other departments or with other disciplines. Keeping medical staff, other staff, other disciplines informed for their information can be valuable. Again, you must weigh it and use it carefully. Gain support from other departments, other disciplines, medicine. There are times when they want your support, and you should give it willingly when appropriate.

Use of the audit process may be a good strategy to identify a group, where it is going, what it wants to accomplish. Groups don't often view themselves objectively, so it helps to stimulate and raise their consciousness level. You, as a leader can play the role of the devil's advocate. I've always said to any staff that I have worked with, "You will never know on some issues where I stand. If I do not think you have dealt with some important component, it is my job to see that the issue is raised."

Last, use as a strategy the desire for accountability. And I do think it is there in the professional staff; I think it can be stimulated; I think it can be reawakened. Many are the times the desire for accountability has been shrouded by our own management styles or structures. Allow the staff to set some goals in terms of the staff's times and standards and allow some decision making to occur on their part. We're notorious in nursing for telling the staff what they are going to do and mapping the steps one through twenty to do it. If you don't think so, go home and look at your procedure manual. We often do that when we are laying out change and what we expect to happen in a department. If you assume the staff should know the process of change, you set yourself up for a temporary failue. You may not lose the battle, but it's going to take you more time. If they know you are with them, they'll move with you and pretty soon they will be pushing you, which is a nice role reversal.

Alfano: With the present value system in nursing, people are most concerned about doing quantifiable functions on nursing units, functions that can be identified as having been completed. That is reinforced when others visit the unit to see what is done asking, "Did you do?" If you can measure it, as far as they're concerned the nurse is competent and efficient. If it cannot be measured or quantified, the nurse apparently has not done the job.

And we wonder why people are task oriented? We measure and identify the tasks as though they are true indices of efficiency and effectiveness. Of course tasks and process are not mutually exclusive. One doesn't do tasks and not process or process and not tasks; they are combined and they do go together.

Our discussion followed a direction similar to others in terms of how does one change, how does one help people accept accountability. One way, of course, to help people accept accountability is to allow them to participate in the decision-making process. I would like to add an aside here. Loeb has been in existence for fifteen years. In all those years, we have always expected the staff to be accountable for its care and for its behavior. In all those years, we have primarily recruited new graduates. I think the number of nurses who refused accountability must be about 0.05 percent. We've had no problem with staff accepting accountability nor have we had any problem with baccalaureate nurses who did not wish to carry out patient care.

If we are thinking in terms of an ALL-RN staff one of the strategies that must be employed is development of a philosophy of nursing. Now we've said it over and over again and I'm not being simplistic about this. We must decide what it is we want to deliver to people and who can do it. Then all the strategies for change that are so excellent and all of the ways in which you help support people make that change become the ways to implement what you want. If you don't already have a formula for it, you invent a formula because once you want to do something, you become innovative and resourceful.

June, it is true that nursing directors are expected to be omnipotent. It is also true that they are usually evaluated as incompetent. So that we have again another paradox about the expectation, and the reason we are evaluated as incompetent is because we are expected to be omnipotent. I have a vision, of course, of Atlas holding up the world and now I have a vision of nursing directors holding up large areas of staff.

Sylvia Carlson spoke about the study of Constance Tiffany (*Nursing Organizational Structure and the Real Goals of Hospitals: A Correlational Study*. Ann Arbor: University Microfilms, 1977). Tiffany went to seven or eight hospitals and used the Verhonick index for a nursing index and the Bell's level of Discretion Index to determine whether or not the practice of nurses in those hospitals was considered professional and whether that practice met professional criteria. Loeb Center was one of the sites she chose and her conclusion based on the indexes used was that professional nursing was indeed practiced at Loeb Center.

I cite this because we have an ALL-RN staff. We do not practice primary care in the sense of the definition of primary care. The nurses carry out and are accountable for the care patients receive. We have had little problem with collegial relationships. As a matter of fact, it's been a long time since I've even thought about the so-called doctor/nurse game. I don't have to play it because the staff plays it. The staff is involved in their interaction with the physician and interestingly enough, the comment I get from physicians almost invariably is, "The nursing staff in this place is absolutely tremendous." Now that's very nice because I get credit for it. It's true that I don't tell them what they have to do and then tell them how to do it, I just tell them what they are responsible for. They have to decide how to do it,which can be even more demanding.

I'm saying that when you have nurses who do have a commitment to carrying out a certain kind of care, then many of the change strategies that have to go on will go on in a much simpler way. We did decide, by the way, in my group, that if you really want a secret kept in a hospital, what you do is send it out in a general memo or put it on the bulletin board.

When we talk about nursing in the literature (and I think Maggie alluded to it) a professional nursing practice does not necessarily define the educational program of the nurse. Professional nursing practice defines the components and competencies which we would expect to find in the practice of a person who practices professionally. When those components are there, we have professional nursing practice. The words I've heard today are power, availability, collegial relationships, principles of change, a process that must be evolutionary (not revolutionary) timing, readiness,support (to explore, to learn, to make decisions), the opportunity to fail, the latitude for error, and then the support to identify and analyze those errors.

One factor we felt important to professional practice no matter which professional group is the ability to analyze what has occurred, to draw from it knowledge that is transferrable to other settings,   to use that knowledge as principles, and therefore, to increase that knowledge. When you have an ALL-RN staff with a broad basic preparation, the opportunity, for that kind of analysis is increased and enhanced, and therefore your staff grows and expands in its excitement and in its knowledge and in its challenge. It becomes exciting to be a part of that kind of setting and it is mutually stimulating, just as the conduct at this conference over the past three days has been for me.

Index